Psychotherapy

Psychotherapy

An Introduction for Psychiatry Residents
and Other Mental Health Trainees

PHILLIP R. SLAVNEY, M.D.
FOREWORD BY JEROME L. KROLL, M.D.

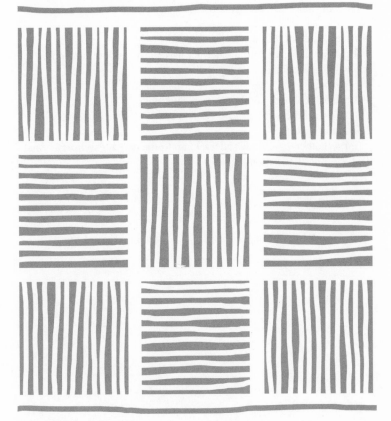

The Johns Hopkins University Press

Baltimore and London

© 2005 The Johns Hopkins University Press
All rights reserved. Published 2005
Printed in the United States of America on acid-free paper
9 8 7 6 5 4 3 2 1

The Johns Hopkins University Press
2715 North Charles Street
Baltimore, Maryland 21218-4363
www.press.jhu.edu

Library of Congress Cataloging-in-Publication Data

Slavney, Phillip R. (Phillip Richard), 1940–
   Psychotherapy : an introduction for psychiatry residents and other
mental health trainees / Phillip R. Slavney.
      p. cm.
   Includes bibliographical references and index.
   ISBN 0-8018-8095-5 (hardcover : alk. paper) — ISBN 0-8018-8096-3
(pbk. : alk. paper)
   1. Psychotherapy—Study and teaching (Residency) 2. Psychiatry—Study
and teaching (Residency) I. Title.
   RC459.S528 2005
   616.89′14′071—dc22

                                                         2004022315

A catalog record for this book is available from the British Library.

For Jacqueline

Contents

Foreword

The Accreditation Council of Graduate Medical Education (ACGME) has mandated that psychiatry residents receive training and experience and demonstrate competence in five "forms" (I would sooner say "domains") of treatment: brief therapy, cognitive-behavioral therapy, combined psychotherapy and psychopharmacology, psychodynamic therapy, and supportive therapy. Is this realistic? How can it be done in a four-year curriculum crowded with competing demands such as clinical diagnoses and the expanding body of biological knowledge and treatments that threaten to sweep aside all other considerations? Is the demand that residents (and practicing psychiatrists) master not one but five forms of psychotherapy a piece of desperate bravado in the face of twenty-first century neuroscientific hegemony, a modern imitation of King Canute's apocryphal command to the tides to cease their movement?

It might be proper for residency requirements to speak to the ideals of training and education, ranging from ethical issues and the basics of interviewing to diagnosing and the medical approach to the psychiatric patient, including all the virtues of consideration and attentiveness entailed in the Hippocratic or Maimonedean Oath. But providing experience, training, and supervision in the various forms of psychotherapy is a practical issue requiring a practical solution. The whole thrust of psychiatric practice is not conducive to a more leisurely approach in which the psychiatrist is expected to listen to the patient, make sense of the patient's troubles from that person's point of view, and help the patient develop perspective, some strategies for change, and a cause for hope. Yet somehow this must be done, not particularly because the ACGME mandates it, but because the abilities to listen with skill and to intervene with compassion are at the very core of our professional existence.

It seems to me that even if many of our future psychiatrists do not plan to or will not be in a position to do much psycho-therapy in the old-fashioned formal sense, the teaching of psy-chotherapy constitutes the foundation of how to understand the troubles and desperation that bring patients to a psychiatrist. Some may opt for a future of computerized symptom checklists, the generation of a coded diagnosis, and the development of an algorithm for the proper medication. This capability cannot be far off, if it is not here already. But this is not what most people want when they seek a psychiatrist and it is not what most young physicians are interested in when they choose psychiatry for their life's work. I tell my medical students and residents that, ideally, at the end of a good interview or therapy session, they should have enough sense about the patient as a person to be able to write a short story about the individual for the *New Yorker* if they had the writing skills.

Phillip R. Slavney's book advances this ideal into the realm of the practical. He correctly perceives that the initial problem in teaching therapy is not to teach particular bits of technique but to provide a framework for examining the very process of ther-apy and to find the features common to all therapies. This primer on the basics of psychotherapy is the natural outgrowth of Paul R. McHugh and Slavney's remarkable book *The Perspec-tives of Psychiatry*, which analyzes the overlapping but different conditions constituting the subject matter of psychiatry: dis-eases, dimensions (temperament and personality), behaviors, and life stories. Each model carries its own theoretical con-structs, methodology, and focus of treatment. The competent psychiatrist must apportion and integrate these approaches when providing care for the single unity that matters: the indi-vidual patient.

Interwoven throughout the fabric of this book is a central problem for beginning as well as accomplished therapists: what to do with oneself in the process of psychotherapy. Issues of boundaries, dress, office setting, and the cardinal role of not ex-ploiting the patient for one's own benefit or satisfaction are fully and richly discussed. Slavney also addresses the details of how to do the necessary pointing out or confrontational (that awful word) work in therapy without coming off as criticizing or attacking the patient. This is probably the rock on which much psychotherapy is shipwrecked, but finding the proper wording, tone, and prefatory words do not come easily. Even this skill is interdependent on the relationship between the patient's narrative and the therapist's narrative, for the distance and discrepancy between these two most likely set up the basis for misunderstandings and problems in exchanges that are less than empathic.

Slavney also emphasizes the importance of the relationship and collaborative work between the resident and therapy supervisor. This crucial piece of psychotherapy training is often dealt with in a casual manner. Residents and other trainees usually solve the problem of a mismatch in supervisory assignment or of an intrusive or incompetent supervisor by avoidance and other pathways of least resistance. But if a resident averages two psychotherapy supervisors a year, a bad experience in this major portion of training seriously compromises learning opportunities, serves as poor role modeling, and can affect the resident's own morale and enthusiasm for psychotherapy.

All in all, this slim book fills an important niche in the training of the twenty-first century psychiatrist. It provides a thoughtful overview of where psychotherapy fits into the overall schema of psychiatric training and practice, and it offers the tools for establishing therapeutic relationships with the great variety of distressed patients who seek competent and professional psychiatric care.

Jerome L. Kroll, M.D.
Professor, Department of Psychiatry
University of Minnesota Medical School

Preface and Acknowledgments

Many psychiatry residents begin their careers as psychotherapists with a mixture of excitement and apprehension: excitement at the prospect of relying only on words and actions to help someone in distress; apprehension about whether they are capable of doing it. In part, their doubts arise because almost nothing they have learned in medical school gives them confidence that they can practice psychotherapy. How much theory—and what kind—should they learn at the start? Do they have to undergo psychotherapy themselves to be good psychotherapists? How much personal information should they reveal to their patients? I hope this book will help residents answer such questions by drawing their attention to some fundamental principles of psychotherapy and to some attitudes and practices of successful psychotherapists.

Although I have written the book primarily for psychiatry residents, much of its content is relevant to the experience of beginning psychotherapists in psychology, social work, and nursing. I trust that readers from disciplines other than medicine will forgive me for addressing the group of students whose educational backgrounds, clinical challenges, and ethical conflicts I understand best.

The book has grown out of my experience as a psychotherapy supervisor and psychiatry residency program director. Its focus is on individual psychotherapy with adult patients. It is not concerned with exploring the strengths and weaknesses of various psychotherapeutic methods, nor with all of the issues that can arise over the course of treatment. My goal is to help beginners get started, and my approach is often conversational, as if I were supervising a resident face to face. I have used quotations liberally, both to let the authors speak for themselves and to encourage students of psychotherapy to read more broadly in the field.

I am grateful to Jason Brandt, Michael Clark, Paul Costa, Chandlee Dickey, Wendy Harris, Francis Mondimore, Gerald Nestadt, Jack Samuels, Martin Schneider, Jan Scott, Everett Siegel, and Jacqueline Slavney for providing information and advice; to Mark Teitelbaum for helping me define the scope of the book; and to Niccolo Della Penna and Anisa Cott for reading and commenting on the manuscript. I owe a special debt of gratitude to Jerome Kroll, Paul McHugh, and Werner Nathan for being my psychotherapy supervisors.

Psychotherapy

I. Life-Story Reasoning

Life Stories

When you ask patients why they have entered treatment, they often describe an unpleasant mood or disturbing behavior. As you ask them to elaborate, your questions and their answers generate the beginning of a story, with characters, a setting, and a sequence of events:

Psychiatrist: What's troubling you the most?

Patient: I just keep getting angry all the time.

Psychiatrist: Angry at who?

Patient: Everybody.

Psychiatrist: Everybody?

Patient: Well, mostly people at work, but I get angry at my wife, too. At work I don't say anything, but at home sometimes I shout.

Psychiatrist: Have you ever hit your wife when you've been angry?

Patient: No, but once I walked out in the middle of an argument because I was afraid I'd hit her.

Psychiatrist: When did all this start?

Patient: About six months ago, after I got a new boss. My old boss was transferred and a guy I used to work with got promoted. He just keeps the pressure on—he doesn't care how the job is done.

As you gather more information, the patient assigns motivations to the characters involved (e.g., "The boss is trying to get me out of there because I won't do things his way") and you begin to see possible themes in the story, themes linked to the patient's personality (e.g., obsessive-compulsive traits make it hard for him to change his work habits) or to events or relationships in his past (e.g., he is reacting to his new boss in the same way he reacted to his older brother). As you challenge the patient's assumptions about himself and others, as you ask his opinion about the accuracy of your interpretations, the developing story makes his distress increasingly understandable to both of you. This shared understanding of why he feels what he feels and why he does what he does becomes the basis for change.

The story that results from this process—a life story [114, pp. 253–67]—is a plausible, chronological, coherent narrative that accounts for the patient's distress. Although life stories are based on information provided by the patient, in the last analysis they are told by the psychotherapist, who not only edits what the patient reports but also suggests themes the patient has not considered.

A Most Natural Way of Reasoning

Storytelling is a very natural way of accounting for human emotions and behaviors. Cultures, religions, nations, families, and individuals all have their stories. We grow up wanting to hear stories and to tell them. In fact, as Fritz Heider and Marianne Simmel discovered [75], stories can be told about emotions and behaviors even when there are none. Heider and Simmel asked 34 college students to describe what happened in a brief film of three geometrical shapes in motion (fig. 1). Only one subject reported the events in geometrical terms:

> A large solid triangle is shown entering a rectangle. It enters and comes out of this rectangle, and each time the corner and one-half of one of the sides of the rectangle form an opening. Then another, smaller triangle and a circle appear on the scene. The circle enters the rectangle while the larger triangle is within. The two move about in a circular motion and then the circle goes out of the opening and joins the smaller triangle which has been moving around outside the rectangle. Then the smaller triangle and the circle move about together and when the larger triangle comes out of the rectangle and

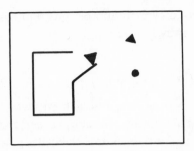

Fig. 1. Geometrical objects whose movements were described in terms of a story. *Source*: Fritz Heider and Marianne Simmel, "An Experimental Study of Apparent Behavior," *American Journal of Psychology* 57 (1944): 243–59. Copyright 1944 by the Board of Trustees of the University of Illinois. Used with permission of the University of Illinois Press.

approaches them, they move rapidly in a circle around the rectangle and disappear. [p. 246]

The other 33 subjects described the figures' movements as the actions of animate beings: in 31 cases, of people; in two cases, of birds. Nineteen subjects told a connected story about these shapes in motion. One such story began:

A man has planned to meet a girl and the girl comes along with another man. The first man tells the second to go. . . . Then the two men have a fight, and the girl starts to go into the room to get out of the way and hesitates and finally goes in. She apparently does not want to be with the first man. The first man follows her into the room after having left the second in a rather weakened condition leaning on the wall outside the room. The girl gets worried and races from one corner to the other in the far part of the room. Man number one, after being rather silent for a while, makes several approaches at her; but she gets to the corner across from the door, just as man number two is trying to open it. . . . The girl gets out of the room in a sudden dash just as man number two gets the door open. The two chase around the outside of the room together, followed by man number one. But they finally elude him and get away. [pp. 246–47]

Two Potential Problems with Life-Story Reasoning

Because life-story reasoning is so natural a way of thinking, we tend to accept it uncritically. The story carries us along as we tell it, and once its major themes are established, almost any development can be made consistent with them. For this reason, it is important to note two potential problems with the method: erroneous information and inappropriate interpretations.

Erroneous Information. If a life story is supposed to be based on an accurate recounting of actual events, then one potential problem is that the information provided by the patient is wrong. This could happen, for example, because the patient's memory for an event has faded, or because the patient's explanation of someone else's motivation is incorrect. Although in many medical settings you can increase the accuracy of information about patients by speaking to other informants, in outpatient psychotherapy you often rely on the patient alone. Not infrequently this is because the patient has troubled relationships with relatives or friends and does not want you influenced by their version of events. Still, if the patient agrees, you should seek information from other informants about the patient's personality and crucial events in his or her life. When patients are the sole informants, you should believe them, but not uncritically.

Inappropriate Interpretations. All psychotherapists have some point of view as the basis for making life-story interpretations [114, pp. 255–8]. Although as a beginning psychotherapist you may think this statement does not apply to you, it does. Your point of view to date has been derived in varying degrees from your experience of life (e.g., whether you have children), from what you learned at university and in medical school about psychological and psychiatric theories (e.g., whether you believe that unconscious conflicts produce "neurotic" illness), from your political opinions (e.g., whether you are a feminist), from your religious beliefs (e.g., whether you consider homosexuality a sin), and so on. Having a point of view is a potential problem because the goal of making interpretations in psychotherapy is to persuade patients to change how they think and act. If your point of view leads you to make interpretations that are unacceptable to the patient, the patient may leave treatment; if your point of view leads you to make inaccurate interpretations, the patient may not improve.

Same Patient, Different Stories

Psychotherapists with different points of view can interpret the same information in different ways and therefore produce different life stories for the same patient. An example of this phenomenon is the case of Anna O., which Josef Breuer [22], Sigmund Freud [48], and Marc Hollender [84] each interpreted from a different point of view. Indeed, a single psychotherapist whose point of view changes over time can tell two different stories about the same patient, as Heinz Kohut did in "The Two Analyses of Mr. Z" [98]. When Kohut treated the patient for the first time, he interpreted Mr. Z.'s childhood masturbation in terms of classical psychoanalysis; when he treated the patient for the second time, Kohut was developing his theory of self-psychology. This new point of view led him to decide that the patient's masturbation "was not drive-motivated; was not the vigorous action of the pleasure-seeking firm self of a healthy child. It was [instead] his attempt, through stimulation of the most sensitive zones of his body, to obtain temporarily the reassurance of being alive, of existing" [p. 17].

You can tell different stories for the same patient because you have to connect events in a meaningful way to have a story at all. What supplies the meaning is your point of view, and the meaningful connections you make are the glue that holds the story together. As you will see in the next section, the characteristics of meaningful connections give life-story reasoning both its capacity to find a variety of themes in an individual case and its propensity to spawn competing "schools" of psychotherapy with differing points of view.

Meaningful Connections

Karl Jaspers, the foremost student of psychiatric methodology, distinguished between meaningful connections, which are characteristic of reasoning in the humanities and social sciences, and causal connections, which are characteristic of reasoning in the natural sciences [91, 1:302–3].

Causal connections answer the *how* question, as in, "How did this patient get Huntington's disease?" Causal connections are established by a process of observation, quantification, correlation, and experimentation, and they produce answers such as: "Someone gets Huntington's disease by inheriting a mutant gene on the short arm of chromosome 4 which contains an expanded sequence of CAG trinucleotides." In this type of reasoning, patients are regarded as organisms to which things happen.

Meaningful connections answer the *why* question, as in, "Why does this patient with Huntington's disease want to have children even though she knows they will be at 50 percent risk to inherit the disorder?" Although observation, quantification, correlation, and experimentation can help establish such connections when populations are being studied, communication and empathy are needed when individuals are being treated. The answers produced by meaningful connections to the *why* question posed above might include: "Because she thinks she will be a burden to her husband in the future and wants there to be someone to help him"; "Because she has always wanted to be a mother and is thinking more in terms of her own life than that of her child." In this type of reasoning, patients are regarded as selves with emotions, aspirations, and intentions.

Characteristics of Meaningful Connections

Jaspers proposed six characteristics of meaningful connections [91, 1:356–59]. I will briefly review each of them, as well as a seventh suggested by Paul McHugh.

Meaningful Connections Are Interpretations, Even When Based on Observation. Meaningful connections reflect the significance of events to observers. For example, a father and mother can see different meanings in the announcement by their daughter that she wants to move out of the family home when she starts attending a local college: to one parent, the daughter's decision is to be encouraged as an age-appropriate development; to the other, it is to be resisted because she is too inexperienced for independent living.

In the clinical setting, it is not uncommon for members of the treatment team to draw different conclusions from the same observation on morning rounds: to you, an inpatient's request for a pass to visit relatives so that he can mend some fences is a sign that he wants to address the interpersonal difficulties you have been discussing with him in individual psychotherapy; to another staff member, his request is a manipulative excuse to avoid group psychotherapy, where another patient has been confronting him about his exaggerated sense of importance.

Meaningful Connections Follow the "Hermeneutic Round." Jaspers proposed that the interpretations we make are determined to some extent by premises we already hold; once those interpretations are made, the premises are strengthened and elaborated. This constitutes the "hermeneutic round." We usually think of the term *hermeneutics* in the context of scriptural exegesis, but it can be used to refer to the interpretation of any text, including a life story.

All interpretations begin with a premise or point of view. A Christian reading the Bible, for example, starts with the belief that Jesus was the Messiah, so prophecies about the Messiah in the book of Isaiah are thought, quite naturally, to refer to Jesus. The Christian reader's ability to make that interpretation strengthens his or her belief that Jesus was the Christ. A Jew reading Isaiah starts with a different premise and so interprets prophecies about the Messiah as unfulfilled—so far.

When psychotherapists propose meaningful connections in a life story, those connections also follow the hermeneutic round. Thus, for example, if we start with the premise that compulsions represent a need for control, the discovery of compul-

sions in a patient's history prompts us to interpret other phenomena (e.g., the patient's refusal to delegate responsibility) as
manifestations of that same need.

Opposite Connections Are Equally Meaningful. When meaningful connections are presented in the abstract, opposite connections are equally meaningful. It is just as plausible to say, for
example, that people tell jokes about their own ethnic group because they are secretly ashamed of their identity as it is to say
that they tell such jokes because they have completely accepted
their culture, foibles and all.

This characteristic of meaningful connections is illustrated by
the contrasting theories of Wilhelm Reich and Judd Marmor on
the genesis of the "hysterical" personality [166, p. 183]. Reich
proposed that "the hysterical character is determined by a fixa-
tion in the genital stage of childhood development, with its
incestuous attachment" and that if oral fixations play a role,
"they are embodiments of genitality or at least allied with it" [143,
p. 206]. Although Marmor did not deny "the tremendous and
unquestionable part which oedipal fixations play in the hys-
teric," he believed that "a review of the clinical material in most
cases will reveal that the fixations in the oedipal phase of development are *themselves the outgrowths of preoedipal fixations, chiefly
of an oral nature*" [123, p. 662].

In the past, psychotherapists often became partisans (and
sometimes casualties) in the theoretical struggles generated by
this and other characteristics of meaningful connections. With
increased understanding of what successful psychotherapists
have in common, however, and with increased emphasis on
practical, rather than theoretical, issues in psychotherapy, this
danger has diminished. Beginning psychotherapists would do
well to remember that, given the nature of meaningful connections, an argument in the abstract can be made for almost any
point of view, including one opposite to that which you hold. The
corrective to this in an individual case is to ground your interpretations, so far as possible, in an accurate history and dispassionate observation.

Meaningful Connections Are Incomplete. Our knowledge of

other people is fragmentary. Many of their thoughts, moods, and behaviors are determined by things of which we are unaware. We sometimes have evidence of this phenomenon in psychotherapy when we make a meaningful connection between past events and current emotions and the patient corrects us by providing additional history that casts those emotions in a new light. Another reason that meaningful connections are incomplete is that some of them start with phenomena (e.g., the occurrence of puberty, the onset of hallucinations) that cannot be understood empathically but must be explained scientifically. Finally, meaningful connections are incomplete because we cannot know the future. Something unexpected can happen in a patient's life (e.g., he or she falls in love) and that event writes a new chapter, with new themes, in the story.

Meaningful Connections Are Unlimited in Number. Breuer, Freud, and Hollender each proposed a different interpretation for the case of Anna O. Given that meaningful connections are unlimited in number, it should not be surprising that more could be found, as Max Rosenbaum and Melvin Muroff discovered in their book *Anna O.: Fourteen Contemporary Reinterpretations* [146]. This characteristic of meaningful connections might lead you to think that, for a particular patient, the choice of one interpretation rather than another is trivial. Not so, wrote Jaspers: "As soon as we believe we can make some definite interpretation, another presents itself. . . . It lies in the very essence of meaningfulness. . . . On the other hand, as empirically accessible material grows, understanding becomes more decisive. Multiplicity does not necessarily imply haphazard uncertainty but can mean a flexible movement within the range of possibility that leads to an increasing certainty of vision" [91, 1:358–59].

A corollary of this characteristic of meaningful connections is that you should become familiar with a variety of theoretical approaches to psychotherapeutic interpretation. One approach (e.g., an Adlerian emphasis on striving to overcome feelings of inferiority) might be appropriate for Patient A, while another approach (e.g., a Sullivanian focus on anxiety in interpersonal relations) seems more apt for Patient B. Your ability to think in terms of various theories should increase with experience in psychotherapy, with supervision by teachers who have differing perspectives, and with your own reading in the field. Eventually, you should be able to employ several approaches to interpretation, depending on the particulars of the case, rather than always taking the same approach, no matter what.

Meaningful Connections Both Illuminate and Expose. The final characteristic Jaspers proposed for meaningful connections contrasts a sympathetic appreciation of human beings and their predicaments ("illumination") with a tendency to see through behavior and reduce it to nothing but the expression of some hidden—and often base—motivation ("exposure"). An example of such contrasting use of meaningful connections is found in the views of Johann Wolfgang von Goethe and Sigmund Freud on why Hamlet hesitates to kill Claudius and thereby avenge his father's murder.

For Goethe, Hamlet is a sensitive young man, dismayed by the enormity of what he must do:

> And when the ghost has vanished, what do we see standing before us? A young hero thirsting for revenge? A prince by birth, happy to be charged with unseating the usurper of his throne? Not at all! Amazement and sadness descend on this lonely spirit; he becomes bitter at the smiling villains, swears not to forget his departed father, and ends with a heavy sigh: "The time is out of joint; O cursed spite! That ever I was born to set it right!"
>
> In these words, so I believe, lies the key to Hamlet's whole behavior; and it is clear to me what Shakespeare set out to portray: a heavy deed placed on a soul which is not adequate to cope with it. And it is in this sense that I find the whole play constructed. . . .
>
> A fine, pure, noble and highly moral person, but devoid of that emotional strength that characterizes a hero, goes to pieces beneath a burden that it can neither support nor cast off. Every obligation is sacred to him, but this one is too heavy. The impossible is demanded of him—not the impossible in

any absolute sense, but what is impossible for him. How he twists and turns, trembles, advances and retreats, always being reminded, always reminding himself, and finally almost losing sight of his goal, yet without ever regaining happiness! [62, p. 146]

For Freud, the explanation of Hamlet's hesitation is quite different: the Oedipus complex—something that explains not only Hamlet's behavior but Shakespeare's as well:

The play is built up on Hamlet's hesitations over fulfilling the task of revenge that is assigned to him; but the text offers no reasons or motives for these hesitations and an immense variety of attempts at interpreting them have failed to produce a result. According to the view which was originated by Goethe and is still the prevailing one to-day, Hamlet represents the type of man whose power of direct action is paralysed by an excessive development of his intellect. (He is "sicklied o'er with the pale cast of thought.") . . . The plot of the drama shows us, however, that Hamlet is far from being represented as a person incapable of taking any action. We see him doing so on two occasions: first in a sudden outburst of temper, when he runs his sword through the eavesdropper behind the arras. . . . What is it, then, that inhibits him in fulfilling the task set him by his father's ghost? The answer, once again, is that it is the peculiar nature of the task. Hamlet is able to do anything—except take vengeance on the man who did away with his father and took that father's place with his mother, the man who shows him the repressed wishes of his own childhood realized. Thus the loathing which should drive him on to revenge is replaced in him by self-reproaches, by scruples of conscience, which remind him that he himself is literally no better than the sinner whom he is to punish. Here I have translated into conscious terms what was bound to remain unconscious in Hamlet's mind. . . . It can of course only be the poet's own mind which confronts us in Hamlet. . . . [which] was written immediately after the death of Shake-

speare's father (in 1601), that is, under the impact of his bereavement and, as we may well assume, while his childhood
feelings about his father had been freshly revived. [46, pp.
264–65]

Jaspers condemned the thoughtless use of meaningful connections in a reductive, exposing way. One should not, of course,
gloss over traits (e.g., antisocial) or behaviors (e.g., lying) that
cause trouble for the patient and others, but neither should one
reduce the complexity of the patient's plight to the manifestation of some repressed phenomenon (e.g., castration anxiety).

Meaningful Connections in the Abstract Are Maxims, Not Laws.
To the six characteristics of meaningful connections that Jaspers
proposed, Paul McHugh has added a seventh [167]. This prop-
erty can be seen when meaningful connections are presented in
the abstract, as part of a theory about psychiatric illness. In this
form, meaningful connections that were seen to occur in the
lives of a few patients are presented as if they occur in the lives
of many. Thus, for example, Fritz Perls wrote:

> All neurotic disturbances arise from the individual's inability
> to find and maintain the proper balance between himself and
> the rest of the world, and all of them have in common the fact
> that in neurosis the social and environmental boundary is felt
> as extending too far over into the individual. The neurotic is
> the man on whom society impinges too heavily. His *neurosis*
> is a defensive maneuver to protect himself against the threat
> of being crowded out by an overwhelming world. [135, p. 31]

An abstract meaningful connection such as "The neurotic is
the man on whom society impinges too heavily" is not a law of
nature but rather a maxim or proverb. Like the saying "Absence
makes the heart grow fonder," it is true in certain instances, but
by no means all. Abstract meaningful connections are useful in
providing concise statements of potential themes in life stories,
but they must not be given more weight than that. The predica-

ments that bring patients to psychotherapy are too complex to be summed up in a sentence.

Narrative Truth

In its first telling, a life story is incomplete—not so much because patients cannot remember everything but because they cannot explain everything. Patients ask for help not in establishing the exact sequence of events in the past but in understanding why they are thinking, feeling, or acting as they are in the present. The answers you give to these *why* questions are framed in terms of meaningful connections between the patient's personality and his or her background and current situation. Such connections fill gaps in the story and enable it to provide a coherent understanding of the problem.

The nature of meaning is such that several possible answers can be found for every *why* question. The best of these answers can be so convincing that you and the patient accept it as true and incorporate it into the story, even though its factual basis is difficult or impossible to establish. Thus, for example, although you attribute the patient's lack of confidence to his mother's sarcastic criticism of him when he was a child, you have no way of knowing for certain that this is the whole—or even the major—explanation for the problem. The patient's parents are dead, he has no siblings, and there are no documents from the period against which his memory can be checked. Despite your inability to prove that the connection is true in a historical sense, if it seems "right" to you and the patient it becomes true in the context of the story. This type of truth is called "narrative truth" by Donald Spence:

> Narrative truth can be defined as the criterion we use to decide when a certain experience has been captured to our satisfaction; it depends on continuity and closure and the extent to which the fit of the pieces takes on an aesthetic finality. Narrative truth is what we have in mind when we say that such

and such is a good story, that a given explanation carries con-
viction. . . . Once a given construction has acquired narrative
truth, it becomes just as real as any other kind of truth. [169,
p. 31]

Could a life story be historically false in some important way
and still be clinically useful? Up to a point, I suppose, just as the
Ptolemaic system of astronomy was scientifically false but still
useful in navigation. Still, both a false life story and a false as-
tronomical system will eventually be found wanting.

When the Ptolemaic astronomers' theory failed to account for
a growing body of observations, they did not abandon their belief that the earth was the center of the universe and that celes-
tial objects moved in perfect circles around it [105, pp. 64–72].
Instead, they resorted to computational gymnastics (e.g., drawing small circles on the circumference of large circles) to preserve the principle of circular orbits and make their observations
"come out right."

If the life story you tell is rejected by the patient or is not helping to produce symptomatic improvement, one of the things you
should question is the story itself. Psychotherapists who refuse
to do this sometimes go through conceptual gymnastics rather
than revise the story. You may, for example, believe that a patient
works long hours at her job in order to overcome feelings of inferiority. If the patient denies it and says that she works hard because her job is challenging and enjoyable, you may be tempted
to say that she is using the defense mechanism of rationaliza-
tion. In this way, no matter what the patient says or does, the
theme of overcoming inferiority can be preserved. I am not saying here that patients never rationalize; I am saying that you
must think critically about the story you tell and be prepared to
reconsider its themes as you learn more about the patient.

This tentative attitude about an evolving life story is important because the use of narrative truth in psychotherapy is un-
avoidable. As a psychotherapist, you are neither a scientist nor
a philosopher, but someone treating real patients in real time.
You must do your best to help those patients understand why

they are thinking, feeling, or acting as they are. In many cases, narrative truth is the best you can do because there is no way to establish historical truth independent of the patient's memory. If you have been an insightful and critical storyteller, what you propose as narrative truth may actually be historical truth, especially if the patient finds it illuminating and "right."

Evaluating Life Stories

Life stories depend on meaningful connections and narrative truth, yet meaningful connections are plastic and narrative truth is not necessarily historical truth. Under the circumstances, how can you evaluate the life stories you tell? The most obvious test is whether the patient confirms the story and uses it as a basis for change. A story that helps produce the desired result is rarely challenged.

Yet what if the story is rejected by the patient or does not contribute to the patient's improvement? Even a good story, if poorly told or overly threatening, can suffer these fates. More often, perhaps, a story fails because it is inherently flawed and leads the psychotherapist and patient astray. In order to minimize this risk, you should think critically about the story as you develop it. One set of standards for such an evaluation was suggested by Michael Sherwood [162, pp. 20–22, 244–57]. Although Sherwood was writing about psychoanalytic narratives, the three criteria he proposed are applicable to any psychotherapeutic life story.

First, the story should be *appropriate* to a particular person and situation. Even though two patients may be anxious about losing their jobs, one is a self-deprecating young laborer about to be married and the other is a narcissistic professional facing retirement from a long and successful career. These patients have a common theme in their stories but very different backgrounds and personalities. These differences will be reflected, for example, in what the job loss means to each of them and in what strengths each can muster to deal with it. The more appropriate the story is to its context, the more it is derived from an understanding of the patient's culture, upbringing, character, aspirations, and the like, the more acceptable and useful it will be.

The second criterion Sherwood proposed for evaluating life stories is *adequacy*. By this he meant that the story should be self-consistent, coherent, and comprehensive. A story gains these properties as you use meaningful connections and narrative truth to resolve inconsistencies, link themes, and fill gaps. The story that results has a beginning (how the patient came to develop the troubles he or she now has); a middle (why the patient's attempts to deal with those troubles have failed); and an end (how the patient's understanding of what has gone before now enables him or her to make wiser choices, have more realistic goals, and so on).

The last of Sherwood's criteria is *accuracy*. One way to judge this is whether the story is consistent with your observations of the patient. If, for example, a patient lacks assertiveness in psychotherapy, he or she might be expected to show the same trait in other situations. If that were true, the trait might be used to explain certain problems and could be a prominent theme in the story. If the patient denies being unassertive, the discrepancy between what you observe and what the patient reports must be resolved.

Sherwood also proposed that stories are accurate to the extent that they are consistent with truths about individuals who are similar to the patient and consistent with what he called "general truths about human behavior" [p. 255]. A truth about similar individuals might be that a patient is easily bored because he or she is an extravert, and extraverts quickly tire of routine. A "general truth about human behavior" might be that grief follows the loss of a close relationship.

Checking a story's consistency with your observations of the patient is relatively easy, not only because you see the patient again and again but also because, in some instances, other informants can validate or refute those observations. Checking a story's consistency with truths about similar individuals can present a greater problem, depending on how you know what those other individuals are like. If your patient scores as an extravert on the Revised NEO Personality Inventory [30], for example, you can be reasonably confident that he or she is like other extraverts in certain regards [112], perhaps including being easily bored [81]. When the similar individual is represented by a single patient (another of yours, a supervisor's, or one described in the literature), however, exercise caution before you draw a close parallel. Even if your patient, like Anna O., is a young woman with medically unexplained complaints who has recently lost her father, whose "truth" about Anna O. would you use as a model for your case: that of Breuer, Freud, Hollender, or another interpreter altogether? Patients *are* similar in certain ways, and your knowledge of such similarities will make you a more efficient and effective psychotherapist, but you should remember that even though patients are alike in some characteristics, they are quite different in others, and that their differences may be more important than their similarities.

Checking a story's consistency with a "general truth about human behavior" can be very straightforward if the "general truth" is something like "Grief follows the loss of a close relationship." Such a statement is not only a matter of everyday observation; it is also a phenomenon that has been studied empirically [97; 133]. Sometimes, however, a statement such as the following is presented as a "general truth":

> Psychoanalysts have defined a widespread, if not universal, fantasy in which, unconsciously, penis and breast are equated; and correlatively, semen and milk. These equations are especially salient in the analyses of those people who have centered their sexual interest in fellatio fantasies and practices, no matter whether they have done so in an overexcited, repulsed, or paralyzed fashion. Much gagging and vomiting of psychological origin can be attributed in part to a person's engaging in these fantasies conflictually and unconsciously. [156, p. 90]

Even if it could be shown that a certain number of patients in psychoanalysis equate the penis and the breast, no data are presented or cited to support the claim that such a fantasy is "wide-spread, if not universal."

As a beginner in psychotherapy, you may be so impressed by the confidence and rhetorical skill with which such ideas are presented that you uncritically include them in a life story—with unfortunate results. If you tell a patient with "psychogenic" vomiting that the complaint ipso facto represents a reaction to an unconscious fantasy about fellatio, and the patient rejects the interpretation or is insulted by it, you may be more likely to think that the patient is "denying" or "resisting" than to wonder what evidence you have to back up your opinion save that the patient is vomiting, that there is no apparent physiological explanation for it, and that you have read or heard an unsubstantiated claim about how human beings behave. If a "general truth about human behavior" is to be used as a criterion for judging the accuracy of a life story, that "general truth" should be very well supported.

2. Personality: The Patient's and Yours

Patients seek psychotherapy because they are thinking, feeling, or acting in ways that are distressing or maladaptive. At the start of the process, they usually relate their problem to a situation they are in (e.g., a deteriorating relationship, impending academic or occupational failure) and want your help changing that situation. As you take the history, however, you often discover that the patient has had difficulty with similar situations in the past, and you begin to see a pattern of troubles arising from the type of individual the patient is (e.g., dependent, antisocial). Although patients are very aware of their symptoms and their circumstances, they are sometimes much less aware of how their personalities have contributed to their problems. Part of what you do for patients, then, is to help them appreciate their vulnerabilities and strengths so that they can avoid trouble in the future and deal more effectively with it should it occur.

Although this is one important reason for you to understand the patient's personality, there is another equally important one. The patient's personality—and your personality—shape the psychotherapeutic relationship, and it is the relationship that determines the success of treatment. (This topic is further discussed in chapter 3.) If you are to maximize your effectiveness as a psychotherapist, then, you must understand not only how the patient's personality has contributed to his or her troubles, but also how it is contributing to his or her participation in treatment. You should be able to adapt your psychotherapeutic approach to the patient's personality, just as you should be able to adapt the medications you prescribe to the patient's symptoms. Before I suggest which adaptations are most appropriate for which traits, I will briefly discuss personality and its assessment.

The Concept of Traits

Personality is described in terms of cognitive, temperamental, and behavioral traits. Such traits are relatively stable character-istics or dispositions [172], so that someone who is intelligent or cheerful or courageous in one situation tends to be that way in others. Not everyone, however, is equally intelligent, cheerful, or courageous, for people differ in the degree to which they have various characteristics. Traits, then, are dimensions of variation along which individuals can be compared to one another. Just as there are gradations of height (a physical trait), there are grada-tions of intelligence (a psychological trait).

The Assessment of Traits

Although differences in height are immediately evident when we look at a group of people, differences in intelligence are not. Unlike physical traits, cognitive, temperamental, and behavioral traits need situations to reveal them. In everyday life, we can es-timate intelligence by how quickly someone grasps an abstract point; cheerfulness by how rapidly someone recovers from dis-appointment; and courage by how directly someone confronts danger. In psychotherapy, our observations of the patient are limited to the treatment setting itself. Although such observa-tions are very useful, they take time to accumulate, and we need to get a sense of the patient's personality from the outset.

Taking a Trait Inventory

The most natural way to do an initial assessment of the patient's personality is to include a trait inventory as part of the history. The goal of the assessment is to learn what the patient was like before the illness began. A good time to ask about the premor-bid personality is just after you have taken the psychiatric his-tory: "I think I've got a pretty good picture of what's troubling you now, but I also want to know what you were like before all this started—what you're like at your baseline. If you were going to describe your personality to someone else, what would you say?" By beginning in this way, you allow patients to tell you which traits they regard as their most important characteristics. When patients are at a loss to describe themselves, you could introduce the trait inventory by saying, "I think I've got a pretty good picture of what's troubling you now, but I also want to know what you were like before all this started—what you're like at your baseline. For example, would you say you're a confident person or a self-doubting one?"

The questions you ask about traits can be phrased in terms of a single characteristic (e.g., "How optimistic a person would you say you are?") or in terms of a pair of contrasting attributes (e.g., "Would you say you're more of an optimist or a pessimist?"). However you phrase the questions, you should ask about characteristics that are important in relationships or at work or school, for these are the situations in which trait-related troubles usually arise. I think the following traits are representative of those characteristics:

optimistic / pessimistic
suspicious / trusting
even-tempered / moody
worrier / carefree
controlled / demonstrative
dependent / independent
cautious / impulsive
stingy / generous
leader / follower
solitary / sociable
patient / impatient
strict / easy-going
confident / self-doubting
unreliable / reliable
easily hurt / thick-skinned
neat / messy
self-conscious / unconcerned about what others think

This list will not produce anything like a detailed self-portrait of the patient, but it will generate an initial sketch. Depending on the particulars of the case, you will want to ask about other characteristics (e.g., ambitiousness in someone whose business is failing, jealousy in someone who cannot sustain romantic relationships). As for traits that are important but may be initially awkward to ask about (e.g., honesty), you will have to rely on your own observations and, if possible, on descriptions of the patient from other informants.

One question that immediately arises about a patient's self-description is its validity. Perhaps by now you have heard an antisocial patient with a history of cruelty say that one of his outstanding characteristics is his kindness to others. It is in the matter of validity that descriptions of patients from other informants are potentially most valuable. Eventually, of course, you will be able to use your own experience with patients to judge, for some traits at least, how valid their self-descriptions are.

Using Personality Tests

Another way to obtain an initial assessment of the patient's personality is through personality tests—either questionnaires that patients complete or standardized interviews that you conduct. It is important to note at the outset that neither type of test yields information that is fundamentally different from what you would obtain with a trait inventory such as the one described above. A trait inventory, a paper-and-pencil self-report questionnaire, and a standardized interview all do the same thing: ask patients to describe themselves. Widely used personality tests can be useful because they allow you to compare the responses of your patient to those of many other individuals, but they are not like x-rays or metabolic panels—they do not reveal things about the patient you cannot otherwise see.

There are a considerable number of both self-report questionnaires and standardized interviews, but a comparative review of their strengths and weaknesses (not to mention their reliability and validity) is beyond the scope of this book. One general comment, however, is that some instruments produce scores on personality traits (e.g., neuroticism, self-discipline) as such, while others produce scores on personality categories (e.g., borderline, schizoid). To some extent this difference is that between tests developed by psychologists, who tend to favor dimensional reasoning, and tests developed by psychiatrists, who tend to favor categorical reasoning. A discussion of the differences between thinking about personality in terms of traits or dimensions and thinking about it in terms of categories or types is also beyond my purpose here, but the topic is important for psychiatrists to consider at some time in their careers [42; 114, pp. 126–37; 183].

The NEO PI-R: An Example of a Self-Report Questionnaire. Many psychologists believe that five basic trait domains—neuroticism, extraversion, openness, agreeableness, and conscientiousness—best represent the structure of personality [112]. The Revised NEO Personality Inventory (NEO PI-R) is designed to assess these domains and the specific traits ("facets") that constitute them [30]. The domain *extraversion,* for example, contains the following facets: warmth, gregariousness, assertiveness, activity, excitement-seeking, and positive emotions. The NEO PI-R consists of 240 items (e.g., "I'm pretty stable emotionally") which patients rate on a five-point scale from "strongly disagree" to "strongly agree." There is an identical form (save for the pronoun used) which can be filled out by someone who knows the patient well [113]. The NEO PI-R takes about 45 minutes to complete.

The relationship between trait scores on the NEO PI-R and personality disorder categories in the *Diagnostic and Statistical Manual of Mental Disorders* (DSM) [5] is a matter of ongoing assessment. A major point at issue is whether the five domains noted above can usefully distinguish one personality disorder category from another [109; 128; 188].

The SIDP-IV: An Example of a Standardized Interview. The Structured Interview for DSM-IV Personality (SIDP-IV) [138], contains 78 items covering the DSM-IV personality disorder categories. Most items are traits that the interviewer assesses by asking the patient one or more questions. The schizoid trait *takes pleasure in few, if any activities,* for example, is initially evaluated by the question "What kind of things do you enjoy?" If the patient lists only one or two activities, the interviewer asks, "If [those things] were not available, are there other things you would enjoy doing?" On the basis of such questions the item is scored on a four-point scale from 0 ("not present, or limited to rare, isolated examples") to 3 ("strongly present . . . associated with subjective distress or some impairment in social or occupational functioning, or intimate relationships"). A few items (e.g., the schizotypal trait *behavior or appearance that is odd, eccentric, or peculiar*) are scored by observing the patient during the interview, which takes about an hour to complete.

The SIDP-IV can also be used to obtain a description of the patient's personality from another informant. In such cases, the informant's observations of the patient are used to score traits such as the schizotypal one noted above. The SIDP-IV, like the NEO PI-R, can elicit discordant assessments from patients and other informants [15; 189].

The Interaction of Traits and Situations

If traits are dimensions of variation, a patient's position along those dimensions determines that individual's strengths and vulnerabilities in particular situations. Patient A, for example, is very intelligent but quite dependent, while Patient B is the reverse. Patient A does well in advanced placement courses in college but is very upset by the loss of a relationship that Patient B would regard as rather superficial. Patient B, in contrast, is quite resilient in the face of romantic disappointment but struggles to pass a remedial course that Patient A would find a snap. What we see, then, is a rather specific interaction between traits and situations in the production of emotional distress or maladaptive behavior.

If specificity is one aspect of the interaction between traits and situations, intensity is another [114, pp. 141–47]. The more vulnerable someone is as regards a certain trait, the less provocation is required to trigger a response. Patient A is more suspicious than Patient B and therefore needs less uncertainty before becoming anxious.

Most patients who come for psychotherapy do not do so because they are in a situation that most people would find distressing (e.g., losing all their possessions in a hurricane). Instead, they come because they are upset by the predicaments of everyday life (e.g., disciplining an unruly child, being passed over for a promotion). In some of these cases, you discover that the patient has coped well with anger or disappointment in the past and you need do little more than help the patient understand the situation better and formulate a plan for dealing with it. In other cases, however, you find a pattern of trait-situation interactions that has produced repeated difficulties for the patient and others. In these latter cases, the diagnosis of a personality disorder is usually warranted and the process of psychotherapy is more prolonged and arduous.

Although traits are relatively stable phenomena, a motivated patient can modify certain of them or at least learn to take them into account when choosing a course of action. It is difficult to study the outcome of psychotherapy for patients with personality disorders (because, for example, treatment variables are harder to control in psychotherapy than in pharmacotherapy), but such studies demonstrate that psychotherapy can be effective [12; 54; 136; 155]. Even without that confirmation, however, you will want to use psychotherapy for patients with personality disorders because you will want to help them understand why they are distressed and what they can do about it—because you care about them. In the words of Jerome Frank, "caring in this sense does not necessarily imply approval, but rather a determination to persist in trying to help, no matter how desperate patients' conditions or how outrageous their behavior. The helping alliance implies the therapist's acceptance of the sufferer, if not for what he or she is, then for what he or she can become" [44, p. 40].

How the Patient's Personality Affects the Process of Psychotherapy

Most psychiatric observations of how a patient's personality affects the process of psychotherapy have been made within the framework of personality types or categories—paranoid, narcissistic, obsessive-compulsive, and the like. In what follows I note some prominent traits in the Cluster A, B, and C personality types described by DSM-IV (table 1) and comment on how those traits shape the course of treatment. My aim is not to discuss every trait and its effect on the process of psychotherapy but to point out common trait-related problems and suggest how beginners can deal with them.

Keep in mind that traits ascribed to one personality type can also occur in another. Thus, for example, both borderline and histrionic individuals are emotionally labile. Furthermore, many patients have traits ascribed to several types. In this way, someone can be secretive (a paranoid trait), have unstable relationships (a borderline trait), and be fearful of criticism (an avoidant trait). The effect a given trait has on the process of psychotherapy will be modified to some extent by the other traits associated with it.

In what follows, I assume that patients with each personality type have sought out psychotherapy or that psychotherapy is being provided as part of the treatment of a DSM-IV Axis I condition (e.g., major depressive disorder, generalized anxiety disorder, conversion disorder). In practice, individuals with schizoid and schizotypal personalities rarely request psychotherapy, and those with paranoid and antisocial personalities are unlikely to do so.

Paranoid Personality

To a paranoid patient, the words and acts of a psychotherapist are no different from those of other individuals: phenomena to be analyzed for their potential to deceive, manipulate, or humiliate. Even though the patient has come to you for help, suspiciousness is so fundamental to his or her way of thinking that the patient must struggle to trust and confide in you. To someone as vigilant and sensitive as a paranoid person, many things are not what they seem.

David Shapiro provides an excellent illustration of the effect of paranoid thinking on the process of psychotherapy in his de-

Table 1. DSM-IV Personality Disorders

Clusters	Disorders	Some Traits Affecting Psychotherapeutic Process
A (odd/eccentric)	Paranoid	Suspiciousness Secretiveness
	Schizoid	Social detachment Emotional restriction
	Schizotypal	Self-referential thinking Odd use of language
B (dramatic/erratic)	Antisocial	Deceitfulness Aggressiveness
	Borderline	Unstable relationships Self-injurious behavior
	Histrionic	Impressionistic thinking Emotional lability
	Narcissistic	Superior self-attitude Feeling of entitlement
C (anxious/fearful)	Avoidant	Fear of being criticized Reluctance to take risks
	Dependent	Passivity Reluctance to disagree
	Obsessive- Compulsive	Preoccupation with details Doubting

Source: American Psychiatric Association. *Diagnostic and Statistical Manual of Mental Disorders, Fourth Edition.* Washington, DC: American Psychiatric Association, 1994.

scription of a patient who admitted, after some time in treatment, that his focus was not on what the psychotherapist ostensibly said but on what the psychotherapist might actually mean:

The patient . . . like suspicious people generally, listened and watched very sharply, but he listened for something quite different from the normal object of interest. He listened and watched only for clues to what, according to his suppositions, the therapist might be up to. He probably noticed every unusual phrase or flicker of hesitation. But, meanwhile, the whole sense of the communication, its otherwise apparent point and substance, its face value, was correspondingly diminished for him. The suspicious person, in other words, regards a communication or a situation not to apprehend what it is, but to understand what it signifies. [161, p. 65]

Beginning psychiatry residents are very concerned about whether they are making appropriate interpretations and suggestions, but they often overlook the fact that for patients—especially paranoid ones—what is said on the way to the interpretation or suggestion may be the most important thing. In the following exchange between a psychiatrist and a paranoid patient who felt slighted by her sister, the psychiatrist wishes to interpret the patient's reaction in light of her past relationship with her sister. In order to begin the transition to that interpretation, the psychiatrist makes a bridging comment:

Psychiatrist: Most people probably wouldn't have thought your sister was ignoring you. They'd have thought she didn't see you when she first came in.

Patient: What do you mean, "most people"?

Psychiatrist: Well, I mean that most people would have thought she went to talk to your cousins first because she saw them first. The room was crowded and she might not have seen you.

Patient: How do you know what "most people" would have thought?

Psychiatrist: What I was trying to say was that there could be several reasons why your sister didn't speak to you first. I'm sorry if I wasn't clear.

Patient: Do you think I should be like "most people"? "Most people" don't have a sister like mine.

Psychiatrist: Again, I'm sorry I wasn't clear.

In this exchange, what the psychiatrist intended as an innocent transition was taken by the patient as a criticism. As a result, the psychiatrist was placed on the defensive and the conversation got further and further from the point the psychiatrist wanted to make.

There is almost no way to avoid being misunderstood by a paranoid patient, but you can reduce the potential for misunderstanding by not making offhand remarks or (what you take to be) witticisms. It is also helpful to preface certain comments with something like "What I'm going to say next is an observation, not a criticism." This encourages the patient to take the observation at face value. Similarly, before offering an interpretation you might say, "I'd like to propose one way of explaining why you might have felt like that. I don't mean it's the only way, but I'd like to know if it seems right to you." Comments such as this underline your respect for the patient and keep your options open. When you misspeak or are misunderstood, a prompt apology or clarification helps get the conversation back on track.

Because paranoid patients sometimes ask to see their medical records, it is important that you write your psychotherapy notes in such a way as to minimize the possibility of misunderstanding. You should also inform the patient when there has been a request for information (e.g., from an insurance company) and ask the patient if he or she wants to read your response before you send it [141].

Another characteristic of paranoid patients that affects the process of psychotherapy is their secretiveness. Their reluctance to confide in others means that they have difficulty fulfilling a fundamental responsibility of patients in psychotherapy—to disclose all information relevant to the problem for which they are seeking help. As they respond to your questions, paranoid patients can withhold information or lie.

Many patients in psychotherapy initially withhold some information, perhaps out of embarrassment. As the psychotherapeutic relationship develops, however, most of them are forthcoming because they come to trust you. Paranoid patients find it hard to trust anyone—even physicians—and may remain suspicious of your motives for a long time. When paranoid patients refuse to discuss a certain topic, you should explain in a matter-of-fact way the reason for your interest and then move on, with a plan to revisit the topic at a later time. Admonishing paranoid patients for withholding information can be counterproductive.

Lying is a difficult matter to deal with in any event, even when the patient does not have paranoid traits. At first, it may be difficult to tell when you are being lied to. As you get to know the patient better, however, false information is easier to discern because it is inconsistent with what you already know about the individual. In perilous situations (e.g., when the life of the patient or another person is at risk), you must confront the patient with your doubts and then, depending on the response, decide what to do as best you can. (In these cases, when time and circumstances permit, you should discuss your predicament with a supervisor or colleague before acting.) In less dangerous situations (e.g., when the patient's developing life story becomes more and more improbable), you should point out the inconsistencies you have noted and ask for the patient's help in resolving them. By leaving room for the implication that you could have misunderstood what the patient was saying, you allow the patient to retract false information and save face in the process.

Schizoid Personality

As a psychiatrist, you hope to maintain a professional objectivity at the same time you convey a personal commitment. This commitment is evident not only in what you do, but also in how you do it. It is important both to care and to be seen to care—to communicate by word and deed your respect for your patients, your belief that they can succeed, and the fact that they matter to you. Most patients respond to your commitment with one of their own, but for schizoid patients such a commitment is hard to make.

The central trait in the concept of the schizoid personality is social detachment, so that schizoid individuals rarely seek out confiding relationships—exactly the type of relationship that best serves the process of psychotherapy. The social isolation of schizoid individuals is not due to fear of criticism or rejection (as it is in people with avoidant personalities) but rather seems to reflect a limited capacity for closeness. Because schizoid patients do not become very attached to you, they are less responsive than many other patients to encouragement.

Another prominent trait of schizoid patients is their emotional restriction—something that characterizes both their capacity to experience emotions and their capacity to express them. This makes it harder for you to know what is important to the patient and whether you are on the right track when making an interpretation or giving a suggestion. Although in the long run you can tell whether you are having an impact on the patient's problem by what the patient reports about his or her life outside of psychotherapy, during psychotherapy sessions you often proceed without clues such as change in the patient's facial expression or tone of voice to tell you how the session is going. You should never attempt to "break through the patient's defenses" or give voice to "countertransference feelings" of frustration at the patient's inertness—such hectoring will only wound a person who may know very well what he or she is missing.

Schizoid patients are less emotionally engaged in psychotherapy than patients with other personality types, but they are not impervious to influence. If you can take the long view and if your goals are realistic (e.g., helping the patient get a job in which there is relatively little contact with other people), progress can be made.

Schizotypal Personality

Like schizoid individuals, those with schizotypal personalities avoid close relationships; like paranoid individuals, they are often suspicious. Because I have already discussed some effects of these traits on the process of psychotherapy, I will focus here on two other prominent characteristics of schizotypal patients: their tendency to have ideas of reference and their odd use of language.

An idea of reference is a mistaken thought that an event has specific personal significance. Anyone can have such a thought, but for most people it is a rare occurrence. You may, for example, believe for a moment that people stop talking as you enter a room because they are talking about you. On reflection, however, you conclude that your arrival coincided with a normal lull in conversation and you make nothing more of it. Schizotypal individuals have ideas of reference much more frequently than other people do, and such ideas are not quickly or easily dismissed. A glance from a stranger on a bus or a statement by a television newscaster can make them anxious and contribute to a sense that others have a special (and perhaps malevolent) interest in them.

This type of thinking has an obvious potential to affect the process of psychotherapy. A remark you make to a colleague as you invite the patient into your office, a new photograph of your family on the wall, a wave of your hand while you talk—such things can be interpreted by the patient as having personal relevance. Is the photograph a sign that you want the patient to marry? Was the wave of your hand a gesture of dismissal? As schizotypal patients work these questions out, they can be distracted from what you are saying or can ask for reassurance about something—like a wave of your hand—you may not even have noticed. If the patient does not tell you that he or she has just developed an idea of reference, you may have a clue to its occurrence if the patient becomes unexpectedly silent. At such times, you can ask the patient whether he or she is wondering about the significance of something you said or did, or something he or she has noticed. There is nothing you can do to prevent the patient from having ideas of reference, though their frequency should diminish as the distress that brought the patient into treatment is reduced.

Schizotypal patients use language in an odd way, so that their speech is often circumstantial, stilted, or vague. Circumstantiality affects the process of psychotherapy by slowing conversation down (and sometimes by exasperating you), but it is a way of speaking by no means limited to schizotypal individuals. Stilted or mannered speech (e.g., using a formal phrase such as "One might say" to begin most sentences) can also slow conversation a bit, but neither it nor circumstantiality makes the patient's thoughts difficult to understand. Vagueness is another matter. The speech of schizotypal patients can be so vague and disjointed that you cannot grasp its point even after asking several times for clarification. If that occurs, you should try restating what the patient has said and asking whether that was what he or she meant. This can be a frustrating process, but the patient is trying to communicate as best he or she can and wants to be understood.

The vague speech of schizotypal patients may reflect, in part, an impairment in abstract reasoning [179]. This impairment could reduce not only their ability to make generalizations in what they are saying, but also their ability to grasp the meaning of generalizations in what you are saying. One type of generalization you might use in psychotherapy is a metaphor—a figure of speech in which a phrase that usually designates one thing is used to designate another. Thus, to a patient frustrated by how long it is taking to repair family relationships, you could say, "Remember, Rome wasn't built in a day." Many patients with other personality types would understand the metaphor to mean "these things take time," but a schizotypal patient could fail to see the relevance of the phrase to your conversation. What does Rome or building have to do with the patient's family? Because schizotypal patients have an impairment in abstract thinking, you should keep your remarks simple and concrete.

Another reason schizotypal patients can have trouble understanding what you say is that they have an impairment in the early stages of verbal learning [178]. One aspect of this difficulty is poor short-term retention of things they are told. To help them compensate for this impairment, you should repeat important information. Whereas with other patients it would be sufficient to say, "When you go to Dr. White's office tomorrow, don't forget to tell him about your dizzy spells," with schizotypal patients it might be better to say, "When you go to Dr. White's office tomorrow, tell him about your dizzy spells. Tell Dr. White about your dizzy spells." Patients whose verbal retention is especially poor should be encouraged to write things down.

Antisocial Personality

When paranoid patients lie to you, it is usually because they want to avoid something; when antisocial patients lie to you, it is often because they want to get something. The defensive lying of paranoid patients is motivated by fear that you will take advantage of them; the offensive lying of antisocial patients is motivated by desire to take advantage of you. Although in reality things are not quite as neat as they appear in these statements, it is useful to distinguish between the lying of paranoid patients and that of antisocial patients, if only because they can provoke such different responses in you.

In general, you will believe that paranoid patients are genuinely distressed and your reaction to their lying may be one of disappointment. In contrast, the lies of antisocial patients will often make you angry because they seem to be feigning distress. On occasion, though, the glib deceitfulness of an antisocial patient is so audacious that it evokes a kind of grudging admiration, which is what Hervey Cleckley may have felt for one of his patients who got into trouble every time he obtained a pass to leave the hospital:

> Several days after being returned by his family from such an escapade, Chester came to me smiling and at ease. He spoke briefly of his plans for the future and insisted on having [a pass] at once. In support of this request he sought to make the point that he had proved himself trustworthy and reliable under all circumstances. Looking me squarely in the face, he asserted with modest firmness, "You know that I'm *a man of my word.*" He repeated this statement several times and spoke most intelligently and convincingly on his own behalf. When I asked how he pretended to be a man of his word after breaking it so many times, so flagrantly, and so recently, he showed no signs of being confounded. [28, p. 157]

In addition to being deceitful because they want to avoid obligations, gain privileges, or obtain money, antisocial individuals sometimes lie simply to relieve boredom—to make something happen. Like other extraverts, they need stimulation [38, p. 11]. There is little point in expressing your anger at such behavior. In fact, it may be counterproductive if the patient—seeing that he or she has gotten a rise out of you—is tempted to provoke you again. You should be clear and consistent about the patient's obligations in psychotherapy—including truthfulness—and you should be prepared to terminate treatment if the patient lies repeatedly, but you should do these things with as much equanimity as possible. Expressing the anger you feel to antisocial patients may only reveal another of their traits—aggressiveness.

Nothing disrupts the process of psychotherapy more than a patient who threatens violence. Such threats are more likely to occur if you have scolded an antisocial patient or refused a request that he or she has made, but some antisocial patients use intimidation because they lack the interpersonal skills to get what they want in any other way. Whatever the trigger, the antisocial patient's threshold for aggressiveness is lowered by alcohol [127]. Unless it is an emergency, you should not attempt psychotherapy with any patient—especially an antisocial one—who is intoxicated.

The best way to deal with threats of violence is to prevent them. Antisocial patients are less likely to be aggressive if they understand that you take them seriously, even though you cannot do everything they ask. When patients threaten violence, you can decrease its likelihood by remaining composed and firm. Although this is difficult to do, it usually helps patients restrain themselves:

> If the therapist attempts to minimize aggression by vacillating and conciliating, the patient seizes control of the therapy and does in fact dominate the relationship in a bullying kind of way. If the therapist attempts to control aggression by

smothering the patient with kindness and reassurance, the patient will likely play the passive role and wait for the therapist to treat him and cure him. . . . [Aggression] must be handled as directly and reasonably as any other symptom, and the therapist who conveys a feeling of confidence and stability is the one who will help the patient most. It would be unrealistic to say that there are not real dangers in the situation, but nothing will cause the patient to lose control faster than loss of control in the therapist. [24, p. 273]

Although threats of violence are the most disruptive manifestation of aggressiveness by antisocial patients, it can also be seen in other forms of interpersonal pressure, including flirtatiousness and requests for money. Here, too, you should strive for equanimity—or at least the appearance of it—as you remind the patient of the limits of a psychotherapeutic relationship.

Borderline Personality

Beginning psychiatry residents sometimes approach the treatment of borderline patients with feelings of incompetence and anxiety. The first of these feelings may emerge as you discover that a great deal has been written about such treatment. How can you hope to undertake psychotherapy with borderline patients until you have read at least some of the literature on the subject? Your sense of inadequacy may only increase as you realize that many of the relevant articles and books have been written by psychoanalysts who use recondite concepts (e.g., projective identification) to explain why borderline patients think, feel, and act as they do. Under the circumstances, you might well conclude that considerable study and specialized training are needed to care for borderline patients and that you are not prepared for the task. Such a conclusion would be unfortunate, because borderline patients can be among the most rewarding of all to treat, even for neophytes.

I believe that, with proper supervision, many beginners are capable of using psychotherapy effectively with borderline patients. If, after a glance at the psychoanalytic literature, you feel incompetent to do so, take heart from the words of Jerome Kroll:

> There are no special procedures, techniques, or secrets which hold exclusively for the therapy of borderlines. The therapy of borderline patients follows the general principles of psychotherapy. One of the basic principles of all therapy is that it be tailored to the clinical state and strengths and needs of the patient. Therefore, the therapy of borderlines will consist of applying general principles of psychotherapy to the specific problems raised by the clinical presentation and situation of the borderline patient. This includes an ongoing assessment of how the characteristically borderline features of the patient have an impact upon and, to some extent, shape the evolving mental and emotional state of the therapist and the process of therapy itself. [103, p. 104]

Two "characteristically borderline features" that affect the process of psychotherapy are a difficulty in sustaining relationships and a low threshold for self-injurious behavior. Even if you believe that, with appropriate supervision, you will be competent to treat borderline patients in general, you may find yourself anxious at the prospect of treating a particular borderline patient because you have already heard about the tribulations that the patient has caused previous psychotherapists.

The trouble borderline patients have in forming stable relationships is due in part to their emotional lability and impulsivity. I will consider the effect of the former trait on the psychotherapeutic relationship when I discuss the histrionic personality, but suffice it to say for now that it is difficult to keep any relationship on an even keel when the other person's mood and behavior are erratic.

Another characteristic of borderline patients that makes for unstable relationships is their tendency to idealize, then denigrate, other people. This tendency, which has been conceptualized in the psychoanalytic literature as a manifestation of the unconscious defense mechanism of *splitting* [94, pp. 29–30], can unexpectedly interrupt the process of psychotherapy. In the initial stages of treatment, borderline patients may regard you as the only person who is understanding enough, trustworthy enough, and constant enough to help them feel good about themselves:

> *Patient:* When I see my parents I get so, so. . . .
> *Psychiatrist:* Angry?
> *Patient:* Yes! I get angry—angry enough to cry.
> *Psychiatrist:* Because they liked your brother better?
> *Patient:* Because they liked my brother better. That's exactly right. Why can't they understand how much it hurt me? You're the only one who understands.

When, inevitably, you fail to live up to the patient's unrealistic expectations, you may be seen as insensitive and uncaring:

> *Psychiatrist:* How was your visit with your parents?
> *Patient:* I don't want to talk about it.
> *Psychiatrist:* Last time, when we discussed your relationship with your parents, we agreed that visiting them might help you clarify some of your feelings. Did it help?
> *Patient:* I don't want to talk about it.
> *Psychiatrist:* Well, perhaps you could tell me why you don't want to talk about it.
> *Patient:* How can you ask me that? You don't understand anything!

The degree to which a borderline patient idealizes or denigrates you may have less to do with your actual qualities than with what the patient desires or fears in a relationship. You may, indeed, be intelligent and insightful, but try to resist the temptation to believe, as the patient does for the moment, that you are the only person capable of helping.

You can diminish the possibility of being denigrated by a borderline patient if you are cautious about supplying words when the patient seems at a loss for them. Sometimes, of course, you will do it and be right (as the psychiatrist was in the first example above), but borderline patients can be hypercritical if you are wrong. Rather than completing sentences for borderline patients, you should encourage them to do so for themselves. This reinforces the idea that being understood depends not on having a magical relationship but on clearly communicating thoughts and feelings:

> *Patient:* When I see my parents I get so, so. . . .
> *Psychiatrist:* Yes. . . .
> *Patient:* So. . . .
> *Psychiatrist:* You get so. . . .
> *Patient:* I don't know. . . . I get angry and sad at the same time, but I love them, too. It's very confusing.

A second characteristic of borderline patients that can affect the process of psychotherapy is their low threshold for self-injurious behavior. Such behavior can take a variety of forms and have a variety of aims. Thus, for example, borderline patients can burn their skin with cigarettes or slice it with razor blades to override a dysphoric mood or to punish themselves; they can take what they know to be a nonlethal overdose of medication to punish someone else (perhaps their psychiatrist) or to bind that person closer to them; and sometimes borderline patients can attempt suicide because they think they have been abandoned or because they have a major depression and are in a hopeless and self-blaming mood. The self-injurious behavior is often impulsive and is more likely to occur if the patient has failed in some way or feels misunderstood or rejected.

Even experienced psychiatrists can find it difficult to choose a course of action when borderline patients threaten self-injury [69, pp. 91–100]. Sometimes this difficulty is due to a conflict between treatment goals. If one goal is to help the patient become more self-reliant, you may think it best to maintain the usual schedule of psychotherapy sessions and to tell the patient to go to an emergency room if self-injury seems imminent. If another goal is to reduce the risk of suicide during a crisis, you may think it best to increase the frequency of sessions or to hospitalize the patient until the crisis is resolved. The course of action you choose will depend to some extent on how well you know the patient, to some extent on your own personality, and, I hope, to a great extent on what your psychotherapy supervisor recommends.

How well you know the patient is a most important variable in judging what is best. Other things being equal, your intervention should be more protective with a patient you have just met than with one you have treated for a year and whose threats of self-injury you know to be expressions of distress rather than statements of intent. Your own personality will also affect the course of action you choose. If you tend to pessimism, you will probably take fewer risks than if you are sanguine by nature. The potential effect of your personality on the choices you make is something you should be able to discuss with your psychotherapy supervisor. In such discussions the supervisor must treat you not as a patient yourself but as a junior colleague who needs advice on a matter of practice. What you want most from your supervisor when a borderline patient threatens self-injury is the opportunity to discuss what to do next, how that intervention relates to your overall plan of treatment, and what you should do if the intervention fails. Whatever you decide, you should document the reasoning behind your choice in the patient's chart.

Try to retain your composure when a borderline patient threatens self-injury. As with an antisocial patient who threatens violence, the calmer you are, the calmer the patient will be. Helping a borderline patient through a crisis and finding a way to minimize or avoid similar crises in the future can be trying experiences for any psychotherapist—but also among the most rewarding.

Histrionic Personality

Although histrionic patients tend to behave in a dramatic, attention-seeking way (e.g., injuring themselves, acting seductively), such behavior is less likely to affect the process of psychotherapy on a session-by-session basis than are two other traits of this personality type: impressionistic thinking and emotional lability.

Histrionic individuals find it difficult to think precisely or deeply about things. What they know of themselves and others seems not only vague and superficial but also insubstantial and evanescent. David Shapiro has described this cognitive style as an impressionistic one:

> Some people search for things in the world—the compulsive person for technical data, the paranoid person, even more sharply, for clues—while others, hysterics among them, do not search, but are struck by things; and what these people see are the immediately striking, vivid, and colorful things in life. By the same token, the simple factual details, the less obvious aspects, the contradictions, and the dry, neutral weights and measurements of things tend to be absent from hysterical notice. The subjective world that emerges in this process is a colorful, exciting one, but it is often lacking in a sense of substance and fact. [161, p. 119]

This type of thinking is reflected in speech that can be almost as vague as that of schizotypal patients, though with a much more dramatic cast:

Patient: You'll never believe what happened Monday night!
Psychiatrist: Tell me about it.
Patient: I've never been so upset in my whole life!
Psychiatrist: What was upsetting to you?
Patient: The whole thing! Everything! Peter was impossible!
Psychiatrist: What did he do?
Patient: What he always does! And Sandra—you should have seen her!
Psychiatrist: What did she do?
Patient: She was just as bad. Sandra and the other one love to get at me.

Psychiatrist: Sandra and Peter?

Patient: No, Sandra and Denise.

Psychiatrist: I'm still not clear what happened Monday night to upset you.

Patient: I felt like killing someone!

Psychiatrist: But what happened to make you feel like that?

In this example, the psychotherapist struggles, as you will, to help a histrionic patient provide more detail and less drama. Your forbearance in this regard should be greater than that of other people the patient knows—and exasperates. As histrionic patients learn to communicate more clearly in psychotherapy, they not only make their treatment more efficient but also diminish a vulnerability to distress in their everyday lives.

The emotional lability of histrionic patients is disruptive to the process of psychotherapy because it can repeatedly force the psychotherapist into a reactive stance. Whatever else you may have been discussing, when a patient suddenly bursts into tears and rebukes you for something you said, the patient's mood and your responsibility for it become the new topics of conversation. And just as quickly as the sadness and anger are expressed, they may be replaced by other emotions (anxiety, excitement, admiration), depending on your subsequent remarks. This new mood, in its turn, may have to be dealt with, and the carefully considered series of observations and interpretations you had hoped to make at the start of the session must be postponed until another time.

However much nature and nurture contribute to the emotional lability of histrionic individuals [166, pp. 100–105], what triggers a mood change during a psychotherapy session is often your failure to meet the patient's expectations. Sometimes the expectations are clear—and clearly inappropriate; other times they are so subtly expressed that you are unaware of their existence. As Mardi Horowitz noted, the role the histrionic patient is playing at the moment, whether "a sexy star, a wounded hero, or a worthy invalid," is designed to evoke a complementary role —

"interested suitor, devoted rescuer, or responsible caretaker" [86, p. 96]—from the other person in the relationship. If that other person (in this case, you) responds appropriately, the patient's emotions will be positive; if not, they will be negative.

When an emotional storm occurs during a psychotherapy session, you can help the patient by remaining calm, even if this leads to an accusation that you are insensitive and uncaring. (Histrionic patients and borderline patients have many traits in common, so the interventions appropriate for one personality type are appropriate for the other.) Encourage the patient to explain why he or she became upset, clarify any misunderstandings the patient may have had about your remarks, apologize if you have made an error, and (perhaps) link what has just occurred with similar episodes in the past. Histrionic and borderline patients who are suffering rightly expect their psychiatrists to comfort them, but that comforting must be verbal, not physical; professional, not personal.

Narcissistic Personality

Two traits of narcissistic patients that can affect the process of psychotherapy are their superior self-attitude and their feeling of entitlement. Although both can be considered aspects of grandiosity, they have different consequences for the psychotherapeutic relationship.

A narcissistic patient's superior self-attitude is accompanied by an expectation of praise or admiration. Psychiatrists generally look for opportunities to commend patients for their accomplishments, but narcissistic individuals expect more than occasional commendation—they expect frequent and explicit recognition of what they believe to be their special qualities. If those qualities are insufficiently appreciated, narcissistic patients can become angry—as in the following example:

> *Patient:* No one at the office understands how hard I work or what I do for them. No wonder I'm depressed.
> *Psychiatrist:* What would they do if they did understand?

Patient: They'd promote me, that's what!

Psychiatrist: Is there anything you could do to increase the chance of being promoted?

Patient: I could do? I could do? You don't understand—I'm already doing as much I can! You're just like them—you don't see it.

For all their sense of superiority, many narcissistic patients are easily wounded, and such patients can request psychotherapy because they have become demoralized. In the short run, they need help rebuilding their self-confidence and self-esteem. As you express your understanding of their disappointments and as they tell you of past accomplishments, their morale tends to improve and they may leave treatment—feeling better, but with the same vulnerabilities. If there is to be improvement in the long run, you should try to help narcissistic patients understand that many of their expectations are unrealistic and that they will be happier if they can be more sensitive to the opinions and emotions of others [125, pp. 421–24].

Just how unrealistic and insensitive narcissistic patients can be is seen in their feeling of entitlement. Many such patients assume that you will speak with them whenever they telephone, that you will schedule appointments at very short notice, and that clinic staff will assist them immediately, even if other patients have priority. These feelings of entitlement may also include the belief that someone as important or deserving as the patient should be treated by a senior psychiatrist rather than a junior one.

When narcissistic patients act in an entitled way, you should first remind them of the context of treatment. (You do not, for example, answer the telephone when you are with another patient or attending a lecture, unless it is an emergency.) If the patient's behavior continues despite such reminders, you should point out how unrealistic it is and—if you have examples—how such behavior has been a problem for the patient in the past. If that approach fails, or if the patient repeatedly disparages your efforts or credentials, you should offer to help the patient find another psychotherapist, for you cannot be effective if you are always on the defensive.

Avoidant Personality

If patients in psychotherapy are to improve, they must reveal things about themselves and change certain behaviors. Because avoidant patients are fearful of criticism and reluctant to take risks, they find these requirements anxiety-provoking. During psychotherapy with avoidant patients, then, your support and encouragement should be frequent and explicit.

Patients often begin psychotherapy without knowing what to expect from the psychotherapist or what the psychotherapist expects from them. For this reason, you should explain at some time during the first several sessions what the roles of patient and psychotherapist involve. (See also chapter 3.) This "role-induction" process [44, pp. 150–52] may be especially helpful for avoidant patients, who are fearful of being criticized for what they say or do. You can diminish this fear to some extent by pointing out the difference between an observation and a criticism. You can say, for example, that you are not finding fault when you comment on how the patient thinks, feels, or acts but rather calling attention to something that may be a problem. Further, during the initial stages of psychotherapy it is often helpful to preface certain comments with a reminder such as "What I'm going to say now is an observation, not a criticism." This type of reassurance is sometimes necessary well into the course of treatment for avoidant patients because their fear of criticism is difficult to extinguish.

A fear of criticism explains, in part, why avoidant patients are reluctant to take risks—especially the risk of changing their behavior in social situations. Group psychotherapy has a potential advantage over individual psychotherapy in this regard because social interaction is a condition of treatment. When patients with avoidant personalities were treated with group psychotherapy by Lynn Alden and her colleagues, the first factor the patients cited as helpful was the opportunity to meet others who had similar problems [2]. A group experience can reduce the sense of isolation avoidant patients feel and can inspire them to take risks if they see that others in the group are doing so and succeeding. Although individual psychotherapy cannot offer these benefits, it can provide the other two things Alden's patients found useful:

> The second factor nominated was the specific analysis of the individual's social activities and behaviors. Most of these avoidant individuals tended to attribute their avoidance and isolation to some vague, ill-defined, innate, personal inadequacy. The social analysis reframed the problem in terms of specific social activities or behaviors to be enacted in specific social situations, thus making the problem a more manageable one. . . . The third factor identified by these clients was the setting of specific weekly social targets and the encouragement to follow through on these targets. Overall, these elements can be seen as a cognitive reframing of the social avoidance and cognitive and behavioral exposure to fearful situations. [p. 763]

In one regard, individual psychotherapy has a potential advantage over group psychotherapy for avoidant patients, at least at the start, because it may be easier for such patients to reveal things about themselves in a private setting. Whatever the setting, helping avoidant patients reframe their problems and desensitizing them to anxiety-provoking situations should be central to the psychotherapeutic plan.

Dependent Personality

Dependent individuals, even intelligent and accomplished ones, surrender the direction of their lives to other people. Although such individuals usually rely on parents or spouses to take initiatives and make decisions, they can also expect psychotherapists to assume those responsibilities. Dependent patients want more than advice from you: they want to be told exactly what to do, not only about dilemmas (e.g., "Should I put my father in a nursing home?") but also about everyday matters (e.g., "Should

I buy a car with two doors or four?"). Until someone tells them what to do, dependent patients are passive—sometimes to the point of paralysis. Although they agree that passivity is a problem, many return session after session expecting you to make decisions for them. And even when you do, they may need repeated encouragement and reassurance to follow through on what was decided.

Many dependent patients take more initiative as they gain insight into the cost of their passivity (e.g., that it angers others), but some cannot translate insight into action. In these latter cases, you should consider adopting a behavioral approach, praising the patient only when he or she has made a choice or taken an initiative and refusing to make any but the most urgent decisions. If you follow such a course, you must justify it to the patient, who is likely to be upset. One way to begin that justification is to say that you will help the patient analyze what goes into making a particular decision, but that making the decision is the patient's responsibility. If you assume that responsibility, you will diminish the patient's distress in the short run but increase his or her dependence and unhappiness in the long run. Your refusal to direct the patient's life is not a refusal of your obligations as a psychiatrist but rather a way of meeting them—an approach you adopt "out of respect for the patient's right to develop" [186, 2:1171].

Another trait of dependent patients that affects the process of psychotherapy is their reluctance to disagree. Although in some cases this reflects their passivity, in others it seems better explained by a fear of alienating someone on whom they are dependent. When patients do not voice their disagreement with something you have said, they deprive you of an opportunity to make an observation more accurate, an interpretation more apt, or a suggestion more productive. A patient who agrees with everything you say may be doing so for reasons other than your brilliance.

You can help patients—dependent or not—voice their disagreements by making many of your observations, interpretations, and suggestions in a tentative manner. This is certainly the best approach early in treatment, when you still have a great deal to learn about patients. A tentative stance (e.g., "It sounds as if you're angry with your brother. Is that correct?") both makes it easier for patients to contradict you and reinforces the idea that they should be active participants in their psychotherapy.

Obsessive-Compulsive Personality

Histrionic individuals neglect details; obsessive-compulsive individuals are preoccupied with them. This preoccupation can make psychotherapy with obsessive-compulsive patients frustrating if you try to point out the forest while they are still counting the trees:

> *Patient:* . . . so I got angry with him. He didn't follow company policy. He knew very well what he was supposed to do and he tried to cut corners. I had to cover for him and I couldn't do my own work.
>
> *Psychiatrist:* As we've seen before, you got angry because someone didn't follow the rules.
>
> *Patient:* The reason we have a policy is so that everyone knows who's supposed to do what. He took advantage of me once before—because he knows I'm a responsible person.
>
> *Psychiatrist:* Were you angry then?
>
> *Patient:* Yes, I was. The situation was different then because we were working on the same project at the same time. We shared an office and he took a lot of breaks to smoke or have coffee—that sort of thing. But we were expected to get the work out, and the only way that was going to happen was if I did more than my share.
>
> *Psychiatrist:* So you were angry because he didn't follow the rules.
>
> *Patient:* He wouldn't just go out for five minutes—sometimes he'd be gone for ten or fifteen minutes. When he came back, he'd just smile and sit down—he'd never apologize for being away from his desk for so long. I didn't say anything about it at the time because I didn't want to have a confrontation, but I probably should have.

Psychiatrist: So he didn't follow the rules then and he hasn't followed the rules now.

Patient: If he had worked hard when he was at his desk it might have been different. . . .

This preoccupation with details makes it difficult for obsessive-compulsive patients to grasp general points—points such as how their rigidity strains their relationships or how their perfectionism undermines their efficiency. As Leon Salzman noted, "Since the obsessional wants to be precise and clear he introduces more and more qualifications in his presentation to be certain the matter is presented in its fullest form. This adds confusion to the process and, instead of clarifying, tends only to obfuscate the issues" [152, p. 34]. You will have to be persistent in helping obsessive-compulsive patients move from the specific to the general, but the effort is rewarded when they come to understand the vulnerability and use that understanding as a basis for change.

Another trait of obsessive-compulsive patients that affects the process of psychotherapy is doubting. Although doubting is not emphasized in the DSM-IV definition of the obsessive-compulsive personality, it is a central theme in the description of the type over time. Doubting makes obsessive-compulsive patients ambivalent, and ambivalence can be paralyzing. An obsessive-compulsive patient usually makes a detailed analysis of relevant factors before making a decision. A number of alternatives are considered in this process, and one is eventually chosen. In some cases, however, the patient immediately begins to doubt that it was the best choice. This provokes a reconsideration of what had been the leading alternative to the original choice, which is then doubted in turn. At this point, the original choice can appear the better one, and on it goes. The resulting paralysis is often very distressing, and patients may drop the matter entirely or make an impulsive decision simply to end their vacillation.

The doubting experienced by obsessive-compulsive patients sometimes leads to a paralysis more severe than that seen with dependent patients. When dependent patients ask you to make a decision for them and you agree because you want to help get things moving, they usually accept your advice without question. When you make a decision for obsessive-compulsive patients in similar circumstances, their doubting often continues as they analyze your advice and vacillate between the alternatives you provide.

One way to help obsessive-compulsive patients reduce their tendency to doubt is by pointing out a paradox: the more they analyze something in the pursuit of certainty, the less certain they become. Although their analytic ability is a strength in many circumstances, sometimes there can be too much of a good thing. If you make this observation, you should be prepared to answer the question, "Then how do I know when to stop analyzing?" Rather than trying to provide patients with a rule (and have them doubt whether it is applicable in all circumstances), you might turn the discussion to an upcoming decision and have them lay out, in advance, what information they need to make a reasonable choice—not a perfect one. In subsequent sessions, you can help them judge whether further analysis is needed and then get a commitment from them to make a choice and stick to it. In this way, they can see whether the outcome of a decision enacted after appropriate consideration is better than one taken impulsively or not at all.

How the Psychotherapist's Personality Affects the Process of Psychotherapy

It is obvious that the personality of the psychotherapist affects the process of psychotherapy, but how it does so is an awkward subject to discuss. For one thing, there seem to be no reports in which the personalities of psychotherapists are described as DSM-IV types, so I cannot use the approach I took in the last section. For another thing, although there are many small studies of individual traits (e.g., spirituality, flexibility, cultural sensitivity) in psychotherapists belonging to various disciplines (e.g., psychiatry, psychology, social work, nursing, substance abuse counseling), the number of such studies is too large and the methodological differences among them too great for me to summarize in an introductory text. What I can do, however, is address a related topic: do psychiatrists need psychotherapy to be competent psychotherapists?

Do Psychiatrists Need Psychotherapy?

The view that psychiatrists need psychotherapy to be competent psychotherapists probably originated with Carl Jung [144], but its locus classicus is found in a 1912 paper by Sigmund Freud:

[The doctor] must turn his own unconscious like a receptive organ towards the transmitting unconscious of the patient. He must adjust himself to the patient as a telephone receiver is adjusted to the transmitting microphone. Just as the receiver converts back into sound waves the electric oscillations in the telephone line which were set up by sound waves, so the doctor's unconscious is able, from the derivatives of the unconscious which are communicated to him, to reconstruct that unconscious, which has determined the patient's free associations.

But if the doctor is to be in a position to use his unconscious in this way as an instrument in the analysis, he must himself fulfill one psychological condition to a high degree. He may not tolerate any resistances in himself which would hold back from his consciousness what has been perceived by his unconscious; otherwise he would introduce into the analysis a new species of selection and distortion which would be far more detrimental than that resulting from concentration of conscious attention. It is not enough for this that he himself should be an approximately normal person. It may be insisted, rather, that he should have undergone a psychoanalytic purification and have become aware of those complexes of his own which would be apt to interfere with his grasp of what the patient tells him. [50, pp. 115–16]

Although this requirement applied only to psychoanalysts, the dominant role of psychoanalysis in American psychotherapy for much of the last century led many psychiatry residency programs to recommend psychoanalysis or psychodynamic psychotherapy for their students as a matter of course. Over the years, the rationale for treatment was expanded to include such proposed benefits as having an opportunity to observe a senior psychotherapist in action and becoming more sensitive to the experience of being a patient. Despite the waning influence of psychoanalysis in recent decades and despite the cost of long-term treatment (even when reduced for trainees), many psychiatry residencies have continued to encourage personal psychotherapy. Thus, for example, a survey in 1995 that obtained responses from 86 percent of residency programs in the United States and Puerto Rico showed that 42 percent of them recommended psychotherapy for their residents and 1.2 percent required it [33].

It is difficult to know how many psychiatry residents have had psychotherapy purely to become better psychotherapists and how many have had it for the same reasons other patients do. Indeed, it is difficult to know how many residents have had psychotherapy for any reason. There have been surveys of personal psychotherapy among psychiatry residents over the last 50 years, but even the best of them have produced results that cannot be taken as representative of residents as a whole.

Some of the problems encountered in drawing general conclusions from surveys of residents in psychotherapy are illustrated in an excellent study done in 1994 by Daniel Weintraub and his colleagues [181]. The investigators obtained responses from 96 of 119 (80.7%) residents enrolled in three psychiatry residency programs in Baltimore. The rates of psychotherapy were 60 percent (15/25) among residents in Program A, 6 percent (1/17) among residents in Program B, and 20 percent (11/54) among residents in Program C. The investigators thought it possible that these results could be explained by the degree to which the residents were interested in psychodynamic psychotherapy and the degree to which the programs emphasized it. The finding that 70 percent (19/27) of the residents in psychotherapy had started treatment before beginning their residencies was thought to reflect the long-standing nature of their interest in the subject. Although this conclusion is plausible, it is undercut to some extent by the fact that 78 percent (21/27) of the residents in psychotherapy said they had entered treatment for personal reasons, while only 22 percent (6/27) said they had done so for professional reasons (e.g., to improve their therapeutic skills). It seems to me that even if most of the residents in treatment (15/27) were enrolled in the program (A) with the greatest emphasis on psychodynamic psychotherapy, the reason for treatment was more likely to be clinical than educational.

It is not known the extent to which psychiatry residents in general resemble those in Program A, B, or C. One attempt to gain a broader perspective on the rate of—if not the reason for—personal psychotherapy among residents across the country was made in 1994 by Sidney Weissman, who mailed questionnaires to 1,442 PGY-4 residents [182]. Fifty percent of those responding reported current or past psychotherapy, but the response rate was only 20 percent, so it remains unclear how many residents have psychotherapy and why.

Representative data about personal psychotherapy are lacking not only for psychiatry residents but also for practicing psychiatrists. The most recent large-scale survey involving practicing psychiatrists was done by John Norcross and his colleagues and was published in 1988 [131]. These investigators mailed questionnaires to 500 psychiatrists, 500 clinical psychologists, and 500 social workers whose names had been chosen at random from a national register for each profession. Fifty-six questionnaires could not be delivered, and 719 of the remaining 1,444 were returned, so the overall response rate was 50 percent. The response rates by discipline were 34 percent for psychiatrists, 65 percent for psychologists, and 50 percent for social workers. Because nine practitioners had retired, the final sample of 710 psychotherapists consisted of 159 psychiatrists, 314 psychologists, and 237 social workers.

Of the 710 respondents, 509 (71%) reported at least one

course of personal psychotherapy: 67 percent of the psychiatrists, 75 percent of the psychologists, and 72 percent of the social workers. It was quite common for members of all three disciplines to have had more than one course of treatment: for psychiatrists, the mean number was 2.0; for psychologists, 2.4; and for social workers, 2.3. The majority of all respondents (55%) said they had entered psychotherapy primarily for personal reasons (e.g., marital conflict, depression, anxiety), while 10 percent said they had done so for training reasons. The remaining 35 percent said they had undertaken psychotherapy for both personal and professional goals. Ninety-four percent of all respondents reported significant or moderate improvement after treatment.

The 710 psychiatrists, psychologists, and social workers surveyed were also asked to describe any lessons they had learned about psychotherapy from the experience of being patients themselves. Four hundred and thirteen (58%) mentioned at least one such lesson. The most common responses had to do with the importance of warmth and empathy in the psychotherapeutic relationship, the importance of transference and countertransference issues, the need for patience and tolerance on the part of the psychotherapist, and the psychotherapist's use of the self in treatment. To the extent that these responses are representative of psychotherapists in general, we can conclude that personal psychotherapy can be professionally useful. Such a conclusion is, however, based on reports from psychotherapists who entered treatment primarily for clinical reasons, so it might be expected that, if they were better psychotherapists because of their own psychotherapy, at least part of the improvement might be due to the fact that they were less depressed or anxious or (for example) had less stressful marriages.

There is a difference between what effect psychotherapists think personal psychotherapy has on their practices and what effect it can be shown to have. If psychotherapists who have psychotherapy are demonstrably more skillful than those who have not, psychiatry residents might be shortchanging their patients unless they undergo treatment themselves. The decision to have personal psychotherapy is no small matter, not only because of the time and money involved but also because treatment can have negative effects as well as positive ones, even among those who are enthusiastic about becoming psychotherapists. This last point is illustrated in a survey done by Norman and Ann Macaskill of all 27 senior registrars enrolled in British psychotherapy training programs at the time of the study [119]. (Senior registrars are equivalent to fellows in the United States and their psychotherapy training programs are equivalent to fellowships.) Twenty-five of the 27 (93%) returned the questionnaires, and all 25 were in personal psychotherapy. Nine of the senior registrars who responded (38%) reported negative effects from their treatment. The most common such effects were psychological distress, marital or family distress, and loss of enthusiasm for personal psychotherapy. It is unclear why the rate of negative effects in this survey was so much higher than the rate of 8 percent found by Norcross and his colleagues [131], but it should not be surprising that a treatment with the potential to help also has the potential to harm. Even if we assume a low rate of negative effects from psychotherapy, and even if we assume that its costs in time and money can be borne, the question remains: is there any empirical evidence that personal psychotherapy makes one a better psychotherapist?

According to Susan Macran and David A. Shapiro, the answer to that question is, by and large, no [120]. They reached this conclusion after reviewing 14 studies in which the performance of psychotherapists who had undergone psychotherapy was compared to the performance of psychotherapists who had not. Nine of the studies evaluated clinical outcomes for patients treated with psychotherapy, while five assessed the behavior of psychotherapists during treatment sessions. Given the difficulty of doing such studies, it is not surprising that most were small. Clinical outcomes were evaluated by criteria such as the rate at which patients left treatment prematurely [67; 117] and the degree to which patients improved, as judged by their psychotherapists [55; 93]. Within-session behavior was assessed by criteria such as observer ratings of a psychotherapist's ability to display empathy [170] and genuineness [134]. Although Macran and Shapiro found some evidence that personal psychotherapy can have a positive effect on within-session behavior, they found little evidence to support the claim that personal psychotherapy makes one a better psychotherapist.

It should be reassuring to know that most psychiatrists do not need psychotherapy to be competent psychotherapists. Still, how do you know whether *you* need psychotherapy to be a competent psychotherapist? If you are an introspective person, you may have already noticed how your own traits help or hinder you in the treatment of certain types of patients or certain types of problems. You may have discovered, for example, that being perfectionistic or taciturn creates difficulties for you as a psychiatrist. Learning how to minimize the negative effects of such traits is, in the first instance, a matter for supervision. It should be possible in any residency program to have supervision from someone experienced enough to help you deal with trait-related problems as they affect your care of patients without making you a patient yourself. (This topic is also discussed in chapter 4.)

If you are not an introspective person, it may be your supervisor who points out that you are less effective than you might be because of a trait-related problem. The supervisor may notice, for example, that as you describe your interactions with patients, you give the impression that you are passive or cynical. If, on reflection, you think the supervisor is right, you can adjust your practice accordingly—if you think the supervisor is wrong, you can correct the misimpression. These are delicate matters, but if there is goodwill on both sides, the outcome should be positive.

However a trait-related problem is identified, if it continues despite advice from your supervisor, or if you come to see that it also affects your happiness or performance in other important roles (e.g., spouse, parent, colleague), you should consider psychotherapy in the same way that anyone noting such difficulties might.

Your personality will affect how you practice psychiatry, just as it affects how you do everything else. You should be mindful of characteristics that cause you trouble and try to modify or work around them. Still, most awkward moments in psychotherapy will be due to the patient's traits, not yours. It is good to be introspective, but you should not become paralyzed by self-doubt. An "approximately normal person" can be a very good psychotherapist.

3. The Psychotherapeutic Relationship

In a culture where self-help books, audiotapes, videotapes, and compact discs are widely available and where computer-based psychotherapy programs are in active development, any discussion of the psychotherapeutic relationship must begin with the question *Is effective psychotherapy possible without a psychotherapist?* The answer seems to be that it is, though only for certain types of people with relatively uncomplicated problems.

Psychotherapy without a Psychotherapist

Self-help materials can be described as inspirational, educational, or therapeutic [115]. Although troubled individuals may benefit from all three types, only materials in the last group present a specific, structured program of treatment. Given the context of such treatment, it is not surprising that most therapeutic programs are cognitive-behavioral in nature.

The self-help programs whose efficacy has been studied can be differentiated on the basis of how much contact, if any, there is with a psychotherapist or other treatment facilitator. Michelle Newman and her colleagues describe four types of program: (1) *self-administered treatment,* in which a psychotherapist does only an initial assessment; (2) *predominantly self-help treatment,* in which a psychotherapist does an initial assessment, provides a therapeutic rationale, and checks in with the patient from time to time; (3) *minimal-contact treatment,* in which a psychotherapist is actively involved, though to a lesser degree than in traditional face-to-face psychotherapy; and (4) *predominantly psychotherapist-administered treatment,* in which the self-help material is used as an adjunct to traditional psychotherapy [130]. Only the first of these types—self-administered treatment—can be considered as psychotherapy without a psychotherapist.

Newman and her colleagues reviewed studies of the efficacy of self-help treatments for anxiety disorders: among them, specific phobias (e.g., snakes), panic disorder, generalized anxiety disorder, and obsessive-compulsive disorder. Although self-administered treatment was found helpful for specific phobias, some contact with a psychotherapist may provide increased benefit for a greater number of phobic patients. The same general results were found for the treatment of panic disorder, with the additional proviso that, although predominantly self-help treatment and minimal-contact treatment can be beneficial, predominantly psychotherapist-administered treatment may be necessary for severely agoraphobic patients. There have been few studies of self-help treatment for generalized anxiety disorder, but both predominantly self-help and minimal-contact techniques have shown promise. All four types of self-help programs appear to have some efficacy in the treatment of obsessive-compulsive disorder, but Newman and her colleagues felt that no firm conclusions could be drawn because of the limited number of studies done to date.

The efficacy of self-help treatments for depression has also been investigated, though not as extensively as the efficacy of such treatments for anxiety. Nancy McKendree-Smith and her colleagues reviewed studies of bibliotherapy and computer-administered therapy for depressive symptoms [115]. Several of the bibliotherapy studies recruited participants from the community who scored above a certain level on self-ratings of depression. In such "depressed" individuals, both minimal contact and predominantly psychotherapist-administered bibliotherapy produced symptom reduction. Very few studies of computer-administered therapy for depression have been done, but McKendree-Smith and her colleagues found several in which computerized cognitive-behavioral therapy was helpful, either as a self-administered treatment for outpatients with major or minor depressive disorders or as an adjunct in the treatment of depressed inpatients.

Jennifer Mains and Forrest Scogin reviewed the efficacy of bibliotherapy for smoking and alcohol abuse [121]. Although self-administered bibliotherapy can help reduce these behaviors, in both cases it seems to work best as part of a more comprehensive program.

The less a psychotherapist is involved in treatment, the more the outcome depends on factors associated with the patient. Thus, for example, poor outcomes are more likely when patients have severe symptoms, personality disorders, low levels of education, and a tendency to externalize the cause of their problems [115; 121; 185].

At present, then, self-administered treatment does not seem to be an effective alternative to psychotherapist-administered treatment for most patients with most psychiatric disorders. Even though self-administered treatments have shown some efficacy for mild anxiety and depression, their usefulness has not been studied in many of the conditions for which psychotherapy is either the essential treatment (e.g., personality disorders, eating disorders) or an important component of treatment (e.g., schizophrenia, sexual disorders). Patients with such disorders need more than information about their problems and suggestions how to solve them—they need a relationship in which they can confide in someone they trust, a relationship in which they are understood as individuals with strengths as well as weaknesses, and a relationship in which the other person sustains hope in the face of adversity. Fortunately, beginning psychiatry residents can easily establish such relationships, which probably explains why the medical students described in the next section were able to do so much good.

Psychotherapy by Medical Students

In 1968, E. H. Uhlenhuth and David Duncan published a study from Johns Hopkins that illustrates the fundamental importance of the psychotherapeutic relationship in determining the outcome of psychotherapy [175; 176]. At the time of the study, the senior medical students at Johns Hopkins had psychiatric clerkships lasting nine to ten weeks. Some students were routinely assigned to the outpatient clinic, where each of them conducted weekly hour-long psychotherapy sessions with a new patient who was considered appropriate for such treatment. Immediately following every session, the student met for half an hour with an instructor (almost always a member of the senior faculty) to discuss the case.

Uhlenhuth and Duncan's study assessed the symptomatic change reported by all 128 outpatients treated by the 128 medical students assigned to the clinic during the academic years 1963–1966. The mean age of the patients was 31 and the great majority of them had "neurotic" disorders or personality disorders. The patients were scheduled to meet with their students for at least six sessions, and the mean number of appointments kept was six. Before each session the patients filled out a 65-item checklist that asked how much they had been troubled by a variety of psychological and physiological complaints in the preceding week. At the time of the first appointment, patients complained most of phenomena related to anger and depression. For the 96 patients who attended five or more sessions, analysis of the checklists revealed that, by the end of treatment, 73 (76%) were improved, none were unchanged, and 23 (24%) were worse.

Although this study assessed symptom change over only several weeks, a similar investigation at the University of Chicago demonstrated that many outpatients treated with psychotherapy by supervised senior medical students maintained their improvement over much longer periods [77]. In the Chicago study, almost all the 249 patients had "neurotic" disorders or personality disorders, and most were seen between 11 and 18 times. The patients were not asked to rate their degree of symptomatic change over the course of treatment, but 75 percent of them were judged to be improved by the students and their supervisors. One hundred and thirty-nine patients were sent questionnaires between 6 and 25 months following their last session to ask, among other things, how they felt then in comparison with how they felt at the end of treatment. Of the 111 patients (80%) who returned the questionnaire, 106 answered that question: 54 (51%) rated themselves as better, 39 (37%) as unchanged, and 13

(12%) as worse. In the interval between ending psychotherapy and completing the questionnaire, only 28 (25%) of the 111 patients had obtained additional treatment. Although the investigators did not provide a statistical analysis of the relationship between additional treatment and symptomatic improvement, they noted that there was a "strong tendency" for patients who described themselves as better on follow-up not to have had subsequent care [p. 178].

In both the Chicago study and the Johns Hopkins study, then, many patients improved when treated by medical students who had little knowledge of the theories and techniques of psychotherapy. What is there about patients, psychotherapists, and the therapeutic alliance between them that makes such outcomes possible? In answering this question I will not review the voluminous literature on the characteristics of participants in psychotherapy and the process of treatment; instead I will discuss some qualities of responsive patients, effective psychotherapists, and good therapeutic alliances that I believe are helpful for beginners to understand.

Some Characteristics of Responsive Patients

Most people who request psychotherapy do so because they are thinking, feeling, or acting in ways that are distressing or maladaptive. They often find it hard to resolve their problems because of conflicts (e.g., desire versus duty) or traits (e.g., dependence) that may or may not be within their awareness. Although many troubled people soldier on for a time, they eventually become demoralized and turn to others for help.

The view that demoralization characterizes patients in psychotherapy was first proposed by Jerome Frank, who (with Julia Frank) wrote that such people "are conscious of having failed to meet their own expectations or those of others, or of being unable to cope with some pressing problem. They feel powerless to change the situation or themselves and cannot extricate themselves from their predicament" [44, p. 35]. Frank and his colleague John de Figueiredo define demoralization as a feeling of distress combined with an awareness of subjective incompetence—a state in which people perceive themselves as lacking the capacity to act or speak in ways they consider appropriate to their circumstances [35].

The Franks note that demoralized patients enter treatment with a variety of symptoms:

> At one end of the spectrum are complaints directly related to demoralization, such as anxiety and depression. These are both the most common and the most responsive symptoms of patients in psychotherapy. Other dysphoric emotions, such as anger and resentment, also may be present. At the other end of the spectrum are symptoms that clearly are not caused by demoralization but that often have demoralizing consequences, for example, the cognitive deterioration of Alzheimer's disease or the mood swings of manic-depressive illness. Overall, demoralization may be a cause, a consequence, or both, of presenting symptoms, and its relative importance differs from patient to patient. [44, p. 35]

The Franks acknowledge that not every patient in psychotherapy is demoralized. They recognize, for example, that patients with antisocial personalities or alcohol abuse may be in treatment because their behavior demoralizes others and that those with isolated complaints (e.g., phobias) may enter treatment in the absence of ongoing distress [p. 36]. Still, they believe that demoralization characterizes most people who request psychotherapy and that the restoration of morale is an important component of treatment, especially in its early phases. Demoralized patients want leadership and hope, both of which even beginning psychotherapists can provide.

Patients also want to be understood on their own terms, even as they admit their failings. This, too, is something beginners can provide. When patients give voice to thoughts and emotions hitherto unexpressed, and when those thoughts and emotions are validated in some way, they feel better. Part of the relief comes from simple catharsis, from saying aloud what was previously unspoken or from owning up to a shameful act, but part also comes from being understood, which is itself a kind of absolution:

> *Patient:* I was so angry with him that I just let him have it—right there in front of the whole office. The guy is so timid it's nauseating. Why can't he just say what he thinks when I want his opinion? I know I shouldn't have done it, but the pressure was really on and I needed a decision—fast. By the time I was done with him, he was crying and apologizing, which just made me angrier.
> *Psychiatrist:* The contract was on the line. Right?
> *Patient:* Right.
> *Psychiatrist:* So your job was on the line.
> *Patient:* Right.
> *Psychiatrist:* So you lost your temper.
> *Patient:* Yes.
> *Psychiatrist:* Anyone in your shoes would have felt the pressure.
> *Patient:* Yes, but not everyone would have done what I did.
> *Psychiatrist:* Probably not. Did you apologize to him?
> *Patient:* No, I went back to my office and took care of business.
> *Psychiatrist:* Do you think you should apologize?
> *Patient:* Yes, but if I do he'll say it was all his fault and I'll just get angry again.
> *Psychiatrist:* Still. . . .
> *Patient:* No, you're right. I'll do it. I just wish I wouldn't get so mad at people who can't stand up for themselves.
> *Psychiatrist:* Have you always been like that?

Although most patients need more than understanding and the restoration of morale to achieve long-term change, if the former are not provided, the latter is unlikely to occur.

Some Characteristics of Effective Psychotherapists

Beginning psychotherapists can provide the understanding, leadership, and hope that most patients desire. What patients desire, however, might not be what they need. It could be, for example, that an aloof and passive but technically brilliant psychotherapist is more effective than an affable and energetic but less proficient one.

There are two approaches to defining the characteristics of effective psychotherapists: the distillation of clinical experience and the investigation of factors associated with good treatment outcomes. The first approach is illustrated by the reflections of Stanley Greben, who wanted to identify the attributes of successful psychotherapists:

> Those qualities which underlie "being therapeutic" are very much a matter of *character of the therapist,* rather than being a matter of his technique. . . . In all my conversations with people who have been helped by therapists, and this includes many therapists and psychoanalysts themselves, none have said, for example, the good results were achieved by virtue of the correctness and brilliance of the therapist's interpretations. . . . I have never been told: "He had a dazzling way of leaping to the heart of the matter, with explanations which surprised and relieved me." Much more often I would be told, "He turned out to be a decent human being who, I finally came to believe, really cared for me, and for what happened to me." [65, p. 374]

Based on his long experience as a psychotherapist and teacher of psychotherapy (including psychoanalysis), Greben proposed that successful psychotherapists demonstrate:

- empathy and concern
- a caring and protective attitude
- a warm manner
- an ability to arouse hope
- an expectation of improvement
- a refusal to despair
- personal reliability
- friendliness and respectfulness

The second way of defining the characteristics of effective psychotherapists has been to study factors associated with good treatment outcomes. This empirical approach has identified many attributes that can influence success with particular types of patients or in particular clinical situations or using particular psychotherapeutic techniques. Among the factors studied have been the psychotherapist's age, sex, ethnicity, personality, emotional well-being, values, professional background, and experience [17]. Within this body of work there is a long history of attempts to identify those characteristics that are fundamental to success in treatment, whatever the type of patient, clinical situation, or psychotherapeutic technique. Perhaps the best known of these attempts is a series of studies by Charles Truax and his colleagues, who found that a combination of empathy, warmth, and genuineness (authenticity) contributed to positive outcomes [173]. Although there is widespread agreement that these qualities affect the results of treatment, there has been controversy about whether they are as powerful as initially thought [126; 148] and whether the research that identified them was methodologically sound [9; 160; 174]. Still, it is hard to imagine that a psychotherapist lacking empathy could have much insight into a patient's problems (save for straightforward ones such as phobias) or that one lacking in warmth or genuineness could sustain a relationship in which the patient is expected to be candid and trusting.

Although some psychotherapists are naturally more effective than others, all psychotherapists can be mindful of the qualities most helpful to patients. If you are not a very empathic person, you can compensate to some extent by listening carefully to patients and by asking them to describe their experiences fully; if you are not a very warm person, you can maintain eye contact with patients and communicate your understanding of their distress; and if you sometimes want to appear as more than you are, you can remember that the role you have chosen—that of a psychiatrist—is best played modestly.

Some Characteristics of Good Therapeutic Alliances

Over the years, the therapeutic alliance between patients and psychotherapists has been defined and measured in many ways [39; 60; 88; 110; 124]. One of the most straightforward definitions was proposed by Edward Bordin, who wanted to describe the concept in terms that were applicable to all types of psychotherapy [19]. According to Bordin, the therapeutic alliance has three components: (1) an agreement on goals (what changes the patient wishes to make); (2) an agreement on tasks (how those changes are to be accomplished); and (3) the development of bonds. The first two components are cognitive in nature; the last, affective.

The tasks of treatment are determined in part by the type of psychotherapy employed. A phobic patient in psychoanalysis would have the task of free association, while the same patient in behavior therapy would have the task of desensitization. Some tasks, of course, are fundamental to all types of psychotherapy, so that no matter what approach is taken, patients understand that they must be forthright about their problems, and psychotherapists understand that they must explain the reasons for their recommendations. As treatment proceeds, new goals and tasks often arise. Thus, a psychotherapist and a patient who had agreed to meet weekly to discuss the latter's distress over a failing marriage might agree to meet twice a week if a divorce seemed imminent.

The process of agreeing on goals and tasks contributes to the bond that develops between patients and psychotherapists, but that bond depends much more on the interaction of two other factors: the extent to which the participants fulfill the agreements they have made and the extent to which their personalities are compatible. A patient and a psychotherapist may produce a serviceable bond if they meet their commitments even though each has some traits that annoy the other, while a patient and a psychotherapist who sometimes fail in their mutual responsibilities may sustain an effective bond because they are well-matched as individuals.

Patients and psychotherapists make conscious decisions about the goals and tasks of treatment; they do not make conscious decisions about whether they will respect and like one another. Respect and affection develop, if at all, in the context of the emerging relationship, and relationships involve unconscious as well as conscious processes. (The notion that personality traits and unconscious processes are determinants of the bond between patients and psychotherapists raises the topics of transference and countertransference, which I will discuss later in this chapter.)

There is a great deal of empirical support for the claim that a good therapeutic alliance predicts a good treatment outcome [78; 79; 89; 104]. This positive association is not a function of the type of psychotherapy employed, and it is found with cognitive and behavioral, as well as psychodynamic, approaches. The quality of the therapeutic alliance is determined early in the relationship [11; 87], so it is important to get things off to a good start. One way to do this is by preparing patients for psychotherapy during the initial meeting.

Every new patient has ideas about what psychotherapy is and what psychotherapists do. Very often, such ideas are wrong. In this regard, the situation today is much the same as that described forty years ago by Rudolf Hoehn-Saric and his colleagues:

> Because of the diversity and ambiguities of public conceptions of mental illness and psychotherapy, psychiatric patients reach the psychiatrist's office with a wide variety of attitudes and expectations. Only the most sophisticated are perfectly clear about why they are there and what they expect. Less sophisticated patients may have unrealistic expectations for improvement: they may not understand their role in the therapeutic process and may be bewildered by a procedure that differs not only from usual medical treatment but from customary social interactions. [82, p. 267]

In preparing new patients for psychotherapy, then, you should explain how talking about problems can lead to their solution. This explanation must be given in terms the patient can understand and should make reference to the patient's complaints. You should set out what the patient can expect of you and what you expect of the patient. You should be optimistic about the outcome of treatment, even as you anticipate difficulties that may occur. The following is a highly condensed example of what might be said:

Psychiatrist: Why do you think you keep getting into relationships that hurt you?

Patient: I don't know. It's like I'm stuck in a pattern and I can't figure out why.

Psychiatrist: So what we need to do is discover what keeps the pattern going, and once we do that, you should be able to change it. I'll be asking you a lot of questions about your background, your personality, and the relationships you've had, and that will give us important information. I hope you'll answer the questions frankly.

Patient: I'll do my best.

Psychiatrist: Good. Once we understand what's causing the problem, we can work to correct it. If I think you're on the wrong track, I'll explain why, and I hope you'll do the same for me. For you to feel better, you'll have to change how you think about yourself or how you act with other people. Changes like that can be hard. In fact, sometimes they can be so hard that you might not want to come in for an appointment. If that happens, please come in anyway—you might make the most progress when you least expect it. I just said that change can be difficult, but I also want you to know that most patients can improve—sometimes a lot—if they try. The fact that you're here is a good sign. Now, any questions about what I've said so far?

There is some empirical support for better outcomes (at least in the short term) when patients get this type of preparation at the start of treatment [27; 82; 108; 168]. Even without such support, however, it is your responsibility to prepare patients for psychotherapy (as you would prepare them for any treatment) and to invite questions about what you have said. As you do this, you will demonstrate your respect for the patient's intelligence and make it clear that psychotherapy is a collaborative effort.

Transference, Countertransference, and Determinants of the Psychotherapeutic Relationship
Transference

The term *transference* was coined by Sigmund Freud to describe a form of resistance in psychoanalysis. The patient, instead of remembering and discussing thoughts and feelings about a person in the past, experiences those thoughts and feelings about the psychoanalyst in the present. The clinical example Freud provided in his initial definition of transference in 1895 illustrates the essence of the concept:

> In one of my patients the origin of a particular hysterical symptom lay in a wish, which she had had many years earlier and had at once relegated to the unconscious, that a man she was talking to at the time might boldly take the initiative and give her a kiss. On one occasion, at the end of a session, a similar wish came up in her about me. She was horrified at it, spent a sleepless night, and at the next session, though she did not refuse to be treated, was quite useless for work. . . . The content of the wish had appeared first of all in the patient's consciousness without any memories of the surrounding circumstances which would have assigned it to a past time. The wish which was present was then . . . linked to my person . . . and as the result of this *mésalliance*—which I describe as a "false connection"—the same affect was provoked which had forced the patient long before to repudiate this forbidden wish. [49, pp. 302–3]

By the middle of the last century, some of Freud's intellectual heirs had greatly expanded the concept of transference. For them, almost every aspect of the patient's relationship with the psychoanalyst was a repetition of past (usually childhood) relationships, and almost every communication—both verbal and nonverbal—was transferential in nature [153]. Because a definition this broad deprived the concept of specificity and obscured what actually happened in the room during treatment, many psychoanalysts refused to accept it. Contemporary psychoanalytic definitions of transference are anchored in Freud's original concept, but they give greater emphasis than he did to the notion that the patient's thoughts, moods, and behaviors are shaped to some extent by what the psychoanalyst does. As Richard Chessick puts it:

> The result of the pressure of [the patient's] internal childhood fantasies is that there is a tendency to reenact them in all interpersonal relationships, always attempting to actualize a derivative representation of an unconscious fantasy. Without being aware of it, the [patient] tries to impose a preconceived situation onto a new situation. . . .
>
> The analyst's behavior or style or countertransference is a stimulus for the patient's unconscious fantasy life that sets off the reaction we call transference. The analyst is given an assigned role to play in the preconceived drama and tremendous pressure is placed on him or her to act and speak in a way consistent with that unconsciously assigned role. [26, p. 95]

Countertransference

Freud wrote much less about countertransference than he did about transference. In fact, he scarcely defined the term *countertransference* at all, save to say that it arose in the psychoanalyst "as a result of the patient's influence on his unconscious feelings" [45, p. 144]. Freud saw countertransference as an impediment to treatment because it distorted the psychoanalyst's understanding of the patient, and he eventually recommended all psychoanalysts be psychoanalyzed to make them aware of the unconscious determinants of their countertransference reactions. (See chapter 2.) Although Freud provided few specifics about his concept of countertransference, historians of psycho-analysis such as Joseph Sandler and his colleagues have fleshed it out:

> It is clear that Freud included in counter-transference more than the analyst's transference (in the sense in which he used the term) to his patient. While it was true that a patient might come to represent a figure of the analyst's past, counter-transference might arise simply because of the analyst's inability to deal appropriately with those aspects of the patient's communications and behaviour which impinged on inner problems of his own. Thus if a psychoanalyst had not resolved problems connected with his own aggression, for example, he might need to placate his patient whenever he detected aggressive feelings or thoughts toward him in the patient. . . . The "counter" in counter-transference may thus indicate a reaction in the analyst which implies a *parallel* to the patient's transferences (as in "counterpart") as well being a reaction to them (as in "counteract"). [154, p. 84]

In the decades following Freud's description of countertransference as an impediment to treatment, psychoanalytic thinking on the topic began to change in two ways. First, the definition of countertransference was expanded, so that some psychoanalysts came to designate almost all emotional reactions to the patient as countertransference phenomena. This expanded definition, unlike the expanded definition of transference noted above, found wide acceptance in the psychoanalytic community. Second, countertransference was increasingly seen not as an obstacle to understanding patients but as an asset. The rationale for this latter change was stated in 1950 by Paula Heimann:

> My thesis is that the analyst's emotional response to his patient within the analytic situation represents one of the most important tools for his work. The analyst's counter-transference is an instrument of research into the patient's unconscious.
>
> The analytic situation has been investigated and described

from many angles, and there is general agreement about its unique character. But my impression is that it has not been sufficiently stressed that it is a *relationship* between two persons. What distinguishes this relationship from others, is not the presence of feelings in one partner, the patient, and their absence in the other, the analyst, but above all the degree of the feelings experienced and the use made of them, these factors being interdependent. The aim of the analyst's own analysis, from this point of view, is not to turn him into a mechanical brain which can produce interpretations on the basis of a purely intellectual procedure, but to enable him, to *sustain* the feelings which are stirred in him, as opposed to discharging them (as does the patient), in order to *subordinate* them to the analytic task. [76, pp. 81–82]

The feelings which were stirred in the psychoanalyst were now seen as resonating with the patient's unconscious wishes and fears—wishes and fears that were as yet unspoken but nonetheless influenced the patient's behavior during the session. Thus, a psychoanalyst who felt annoyed while a patient spoke critically of her mother might subsequently link that feeling to the patient's narcissistic desire for praise. Countertransference was thought to reveal important information not only about the nature of the patient's unconscious feelings but also about the degree of the patient's regression, so that "the more intense and premature the therapist's emotional reaction to the patient, the more threatening it becomes to the therapist's neutrality . . . the more we can think the therapist is in the presence of severe regression in the patient" [95, p. 43].

Although many psychotherapists do not find the psychoanalytic concept of regression useful, they do believe that emotions provoked by a patient's verbal and nonverbal communications can provide hints to the patient's underlying psychological state. (It is, of course, essential to regard such hints *as* hints, rather than facts, lest you fall into the trap of believing that your "gut feelings" are an infallible source of information about the patient—something a psychoanalyst would warn against.)

Just as contemporary students of transference such as Richard Chessick (see above) invoke countertransference to explain what they mean by the concept that interests them, so contemporary students of countertransference such as Glen Gabbard invoke transference to explain what they mean by the concept that interests *them*:

> Today, clinicians of all persuasions generally accept the idea that countertransference can be a useful source of information about the patient. At the same time, the therapist's own subjectivity is involved in the way the patient's behavior is experienced. Hence, there is a movement in the direction of regarding countertransference as a *jointly created* phenomenon that involves contributions from both patient and clinician. The patient draws the therapist into playing a role that reflects the patient's internal world, but the specific dimensions of that role are colored by the therapist's own personality. [52, p. 984]

Determinants of the Psychotherapeutic Relationship

For all that has been written about transference and countertransference, they are not the major determinants of the psychotherapeutic relationship. Other factors are more important, both because they operate earlier in the relationship and because they are more fundamental to it. In my view, those factors are the social roles of patient and psychotherapist, the treatment approach used by the psychotherapist, and the personalities of the patient and the psychotherapist.

To be a patient, a psychotherapist, a parent, a teacher, a soldier, or a priest is to occupy a certain social role. Each role is characterized by a set of attitudes and behaviors that are expected of its occupant. Thus, for example, patients are expected to regard illness as an undesirable state and to cooperate with physicians and others who try to help them get well, while physicians are expected to regard their patients as worthy of help and to refrain from exploiting them. Although most people are quite familiar with the attitudes and behaviors expected of patients in general, those expected of patients in psychotherapy are less familiar, which is why it is important to prepare patients for treatment in the manner described above. In a similar way, although by now you are quite familiar with the attitudes and behaviors expected of physicians in general, those expected of you as a psychotherapist are less familiar, which is why it is important for you to have supervision. All psychotherapeutic relationships are grounded in the social roles of the participants, a fact that becomes especially—sometimes painfully—obvious when the boundaries of those roles are transgressed. (See below for a discussion of the boundaries of the psychotherapeutic relationship.)

A second major factor determining the psychotherapeutic relationship is the treatment approach adopted by the psychotherapist. Do you ask about the patient's fantasies or not? Are you on a first-name basis with the patient or not? Do you use hypnosis or not? Do you ask the patient to sit in a chair or lie on a couch? Do you touch the patient or not? These are more than technical questions; their answers determine whether certain types of thoughts and actions are discouraged, tolerated, or promoted.

Although Sigmund Freud sat behind his reclining patients because he could not stand being stared at for eight hours a day, he also did it to avoid contaminating their transference reactions: "Since, while I am listening to the patient, I, too, give myself over to the current of my unconscious thoughts, I do not wish my expressions of face to give the patient material for interpretations or to influence him in what he tells me. The patient usually regards being made to adopt this position as a hardship and rebels against it. . . . I insist on this procedure, however, for its purpose and result are to prevent the transference from mingling with the patient's associations imperceptibly, to isolate the transference and to allow it to come forward in due course sharply defined as a resistance" [47, p. 134]. This psychoanalytic technique fosters a very different type of relationship between the psychotherapist and the patient than the Gestalt technique developed by Fritz Perls:

In this model, the therapist is available for work with one person . . . at a time. The volunteer client takes the "hot seat" facing the therapist, sometimes in the center of the group and sometimes in the circle of group members. While the therapist and client explore whatever phenomena emerge in their interaction, the rest of the group members remain silent and are spectators, not unlike the Greek choruses who replied to or commented on the dramatic action in the play. Although limited, the chorus performed an essential function, as does the group in Gestalt therapy. At certain points the group may be called into action by the therapist, but usually this is done in a structured way to further the client's work. . . .

The controlling factor in the client's interaction with the group members is the therapist's intention to keep the focus on the client and to encourage that person to take responsibility for his or her own experience. [99, pp. 105–6]

The treatment approach you adopt provides a script for you and the patient to follow. It decides, to a greater or lesser degree, how the two of you interact, which words you use when speaking to one another, and what constitutes a good performance. The social roles of the psychotherapist and the patient determine the general character of their relationship; the treatment approach gives those roles more definition.

Personality is the third major factor determining the nature of the psychotherapeutic relationship. The less doctrinaire your treatment approach, the more your personality and that of your patient shape the expression of your social roles and the affective component of the therapeutic alliance. Even if you stick to the script of a single therapeutic method, your relationship with patients will differ to the extent that they are dependent or independent, trusting or suspicious, impertinent or respectful. In the same way, their response to you will vary to the degree that you are controlling or permissive, jocular or solemn, predictable or erratic.

Every now and then a patient or a psychotherapist does something out of character and their relationship suffers. One reason for such occurrences is the displacement of feelings from another relationship or situation—not in the sense of transference or countertransference (in the Freudian meaning of the latter term), but in the sense that you might be irritable with Patient A because ten minutes earlier you were insulted by Patient B. If this happens, an apology from the offending party should set matters right.

Another reason that patients or psychotherapists sometimes act out of character is that they are intoxicated or have developed an illness such as depression or mania. If a patient is intoxicated, you should abort the session with a reminder that psychotherapy requires concentration and reflection. Intoxication in a psychotherapist is more serious than intoxication in a patient. A psychotherapist who is intoxicated ipso facto has poor judgment. That psychotherapist also has difficulty concentrating and therefore difficulty thinking through complicated issues—exactly the type of thinking a patient has every right to expect. If you attempt to practice psychotherapy while intoxicated, you violate the patient's trust. Rather than risk harm to the patient, you must cancel the session. If you are intoxicated more than once, you must suspend your practice and obtain treatment.

When patients develop severe depression or mania, the cause of their uncharacteristic behavior is obvious; when the affective disorder is mild, however, it might take several sessions for you to realize what is happening. You can make the diagnosis more quickly if you do a mental status examination whenever there is an unexpected change in a patient's mood, thinking, or behavior, especially if it persists from session to session. Stepping back from the flow of psychotherapy can help you see that, although Patient A *might* be irritable because she is ambivalent about what you are asking her to do or Patient B *might* be taciturn because he is having a transference reaction, the correct explanation for their uncharacteristic behavior is that each has developed an affective disorder.

When psychotherapists become severely depressed, they usually feel ill, doubt their abilities, have difficulty concentrating, and lose the drive to work. For these reasons, they often stop seeing patients and enter treatment, either on their own—especially if they have been depressed in the past and recognize a relapse—or with encouragement from family members or colleagues. When psychotherapists become severely manic, however, they usually do not see themselves as ill and they resist the advice of relatives and colleagues to consult a psychiatrist, even if they have been manic before. Like other people with severe mania, they usually have great confidence in their abilities despite the fact that their thinking is disorganized, and they can do a great deal of harm to themselves and others—including their patients—if they are irritable or hypersexual.

Although psychotherapists with mild affective disorders often continue to work, their illness can damage their relationship with their patients. If a depressed psychotherapist is apathetic, for example, a patient who needs encouragement may not get it. And if a hypomanic psychotherapist is condescending, a patient with low self-esteem may feel even more debased. If you ever wonder whether you have an affective disorder, or if a relative or colleague raises the question, you owe it to your patients, your family, and yourself to take the matter seriously.

Finally, patients and psychotherapists can act out of character because they are having transference and countertransference reactions, respectively. (Here I am using *countertransference* in the Freudian sense.) When this occurs, the emotions expressed are intense and inappropriate to the situation. If you suspect a transference or countertransference reaction, discuss your observations with your psychotherapy supervisor, who should be able help you identify the phenomenon and deal with it.

The Boundaries of the Psychotherapeutic Relationship

Although you may have affectionate—even amorous—feelings for your patients, you must not encourage them to become your lovers. Although you use the psychotherapeutic relationship to help patients overcome their problems, you must not use it to help overcome your own. And although you gain monetarily from the care you provide, you must not exploit your patients financially. If you do these things, you violate the boundaries of the psychotherapeutic relationship and the trust your patients have placed in you.

People become psychotherapists to help others, not to harm them, so why do some psychotherapists act unethically? One reason is that their judgment is impaired by intoxication or a disorder such as depression or mania. When this occurs, the affected psychotherapist can show poor judgment about many things in both professional and nonprofessional relationships. (In the rare case of psychotherapists with paraphilic disorders, the impairment of judgment is much more restricted in scope.) Another reason psychotherapists can act unethically is that, despite the values instilled by their professional education—and sometimes despite their personal psychotherapy—they yield to antisocial, borderline, histrionic, narcissistic, or dependent traits when their nonprofessional relationships are unsatisfactory or when (as sometimes occurs) a patient entices them. A final reason is that psychotherapists, whatever their personalities, can deceive themselves into thinking that they are acting in their patients' interest rather than their own [51]. Such self-deceptions may be especially common in sexual misconduct.

Sexual Misconduct

According to Robert Simon, there is a fairly typical sequence of events in sexual misconduct by psychotherapists [164]. The sequence may begin when the psychotherapist and the patient start to address one another by their first names. After that, their sessions become increasingly social in nature and the psychotherapist reveals more and more about his or her own feelings and interests. In due course the sessions, which used to end verbally, terminate with a handshake and then with a hug. Eventually, sessions are scheduled for the end of the day, after which the couple begin to have dinner with each other and, perhaps, see a movie together. Hand-holding, kissing, and intercourse follow in their turns. Simon identifies the time "between the chair and the door" as an especially dangerous transition in this sequence [165], but it is easy to understand how each transition could lower the threshold for the following one.

Thomas Gutheil and Glen Gabbard described this process as a "slippery slope" [71; 72]. In doing so, they indicated both the gradual nature of the descent into misconduct and the difficulty a psychotherapist can have in stopping it. Jerome Kroll criticizes the notion of a slippery slope on empirical and conceptual grounds [102]. Kroll wants to know, for example, how often psychotherapists and patients who address each other by their first names actually proceed to sexual intercourse. He insists that the earliest acts in the sequence described by Simon—the use of first names and limited self-disclosure by psychotherapists—are perfectly acceptable techniques in certain treatment methods and therefore do not ipso facto represent crossings of the boundary between a professional and a personal relationship. Kroll identifies the slippery-slope argument as a post hoc one— a point also made by Ofer Zur and Arnold Lazarus: "To assert that self-disclosure, a hug, a home visit, or accepting a gift are actions likely to lead to sex is like saying that doctors' visits cause death because most people see a doctor before they die" [190, p. 9].

Gutheil, Gabbard, and Simon responded to such criticisms by (among other things) reiterating their acknowledgment that techniques appropriate in one treatment method might not be appropriate in another [51; 73; 163]. Thus, for example, "a behavior therapist assisting an agoraphobic patient through use of in vivo exposure may drive the patient to a shopping mall to encounter the feared situation. A clinician engaged in psychoanalytic psychotherapy would be in serious need of supervision if similar activities were going on. Even within psychodynamic therapy, however, the appropriate frame varies from patient to patient. Certain patients require greater degrees of verbal activity or therapeutic self-disclosure for them to feel engaged in a treatment process. Also, some therapists may have a more self-revelatory style than others" [71, pp. 411–12]. Gutheil, Gabbard, and Simon allow for variations in treatment technique and personal style, but their experience evaluating and treating psychotherapists who commit sexual misconduct leads them to conclude that the unethical behavior often begins with a series of apparently harmless acts.

How Many Psychotherapists Find Their Patients Attractive? It is reasonable to assume that the number of psychotherapists who find their patients sexually attractive is much greater than the number who commit sexual misconduct. To my knowledge, only one study has tested that assumption. The study was published in 1986 by Kenneth Pope and his colleagues, who tried to ascertain how many psychologists found their patients attractive and what they found attractive about them [139]. The investigators sent an anonymous questionnaire to 500 male and 500 female psychologists randomly selected from the 4,356 members of the American Psychological Association's division for psychologists in private practice. Of the 1,000 potential respondents, 585 (58.5%) returned the questionnaire, and of these, 339 (57.9%) were men and 246 (42.1%) were women. Almost half (48.9%) of the respondents were between the ages of 30 and 45; 39.0 percent were between 46 and 60; and 12.1 percent were over 60. As a group, they averaged 16.9 years of professional experience.

Five hundred and eight of the 585 respondents (86.8%) reported being attracted to at least one patient, with 322 (94.9%) of the men and 186 (75.6%) of the women acknowledging such feelings. When asked in an open-ended question what it was about their patients they had found attractive, the respondents answered with 997 descriptive terms, which the investigators sorted into 19 categories. The largest category (296 responses) was physical attractiveness, which included terms such as *beautiful* and *athletic*. The next largest category (124 responses) was intellectual attractiveness, which included terms such as *intelligent* and *articulate*. The third-largest (88 responses) was sexual attractiveness, which not only included terms such as *sexy* but also notations that sexual material was discussed during psychotherapy, while the fourth-largest (85 responses) had to do with the patient's vulnerabilities, as indicated by terms such as *childlike* and *sensitive*.

Although the vast majority of psychologists surveyed had

found some patients attractive for one reason or another, 93.5 percent said they had never been sexually intimate with their patients. (What constituted sexual intimacy was not defined in the paper.) Among the 6.5 percent of respondents who acknowledged sexual intimacy with patients, the rate was higher among men (9.4%) than women (2.5%). Most respondents (57.0%) who were sexually attracted to patients sought supervision or consultation about their feelings—a practice that was more common among younger psychologists than older ones but equally common among males and females.

The psychologists who reported having been attracted to patients without becoming sexually involved gave a variety of reasons for their abstinence. The open-ended question that assessed this topic generated 1,091 responses, which the investigators sorted into 14 categories. The largest category (289 responses) was that sexual involvement with patients was unethical. The next largest were that it was countertherapeutic or exploitative (251 responses), unprofessional (134 responses), or against the respondent's personal values (133 responses).

Although the study by Pope and his colleagues is a valuable one, it faces two methodological questions that confront all self-report surveys: (1) Is the sample representative? and (2) Are the responses valid? The latter question may be especially important when the topic of the survey is a stigmatized behavior such as sexual misconduct or substance abuse. One indication of the potential gap between what people report they do and what they actually do can be found in a 1992 survey sent by John Lamont and Christel Woodward to all 792 members of the Society of Obstetricians and Gynaecologists of Canada [106]. Six hundred and eighteen (78.0%) members responded, and of these, 497 (80.4%) were male and 121 (19.6%) were female. The average age of the respondents was 47.3 years and their average time in practice was 16.8 years. Of this sample, 3 percent of the males and 1 percent of the females acknowledged sexual involvement (according to the respondent's own definition of that phrase) with someone who was a patient at the time. In contrast, 17 percent of females and 8 percent of males reported knowing that a colleague in obstetrics and gynecology had been involved with a current patient. Although it is possible that the latter figures could overestimate the frequency of sexual misconduct by Canadian obstetricians and gynecologists if several respondents were aware of the same colleague's behavior, my point here is that the actual rate of sexual misconduct in any group is almost certainly higher than the rate derived from self-reports.

Methodological issues notwithstanding, anonymous self-report surveys have been the most common way of estimating the frequency of sexual misconduct by physicians in general, by practicing psychiatrists, and by psychiatry residents. What do such surveys reveal?

How Common Is Sexual Misconduct by Physicians in General? If the Hippocratic Oath is any indication, sexual misconduct by physicians has been a problem for thousands of years. In the traditional version of the Oath, physicians swear to "come for the benefit of the sick, remaining free of all intentional injustice, of all mischief and in particular of sexual relations with both female and male persons, be they free or slave" [37, p. 3]. Despite this and similar prohibitions over the centuries, and despite the principle of *primum non nocere ("first, do no harm")*, physicians have continued to engage in sexual misconduct.

Table 2 summarizes the results of eight surveys of physicians in various specialties about their sexual involvement with current or former patients. Although the studies differ in how they defined and asked about sexual involvement, in the size and diversity of the groups they sampled, and in the response rates they achieved, all of them discovered some physicians who were willing to acknowledge (and in some cases to defend as therapeutic) behaviors that ranged from touching for the purpose of sexual arousal to intercourse. The rates of sexual involvement differed from study to study for a given specialty (e.g., 3 to 10 percent for obstetrics and gynecology), but considering all of the studies, the rates were roughly comparable from one specialty to another. In the six surveys that included both male and female physicians, the rates for sexual involvement were consistently higher for males. If we assume that the actual rate of sexual mis-

Table 2. Surveys of Sexual Misconduct by Physicians

Authors; Publication Date	Physicians Surveyed	Number and Source	Sex of Respondents	Response Rate (%)	Overall Rate of Sexual Involvement with Patients (%)
Kardener et al. 1973 [92]	Fam Prac, Int Med Ob-Gyn, Psych, Surg	1,000 randomly selected from county medical society	Male	46	12.8
Perry 1976 [137]	Fam Prac, Int Med, Ped, Psych, Other	500 randomly selected from NY and CA	Female	31	0.6
Wilbers et al. 1992 [184]	Ob-Gyn, Otol	All 975 members of both Dutch specialty societies	Both	67	4
Gartrell et al. 1992 [58]	Fam Prac, Int Med, Ob-Gyn, Surg	10,000 randomly selected from AMA Physician Masterfile	Both	19	9

Lamont and Woodward 1994 [106]	Ob-Gyn	All 792 members of Society of Obstetricians and Gynaecologists of Canada	Both	78	3
Coverdale et al. 1995 [32]	Fam Prac	217 randomly selected from all New Zealand family practitioners	Both	86.2	3.8
Bayer et al. 1996 [13]	Fam Prac, Int Med, Ob-Gyn, Ophth	1,600 randomly selected from AMA Physician Masterfile	Both	52	3.4
Ovens and Permaul-Woods 1997 [132]	Emg Med	974 from commercial mailing list in Ontario, Canada	Both	61.5	6.2

Abbreviations: AMA = American Medical Association; Emg Med = Emergency Medicine; Fam Prac = Family Practice; Int Med = Internal Medicine; Ob-Gyn = Obstetrics and Gynecology; Ophth = Ophthalmology; Otol = Otolaryngology; Ped = Pediatrics; Psych = Psychiatry; Surg = Surgery conduct is greater than the lowest rates acknowledged in these surveys, then some 5 to 10 percent of male physicians have adulterated the doctor-patient relationship.

How Common Is Sexual Misconduct by Practicing Psychiatrists? Table 3 summarizes the results of three surveys of practicing psychiatrists about their sexual involvement with current or former patients. (The survey by Judith Perry listed in table 2 is not included because it does not give response rates by specialty. None of the 30 female psychiatrists in that study acknowledged sexual involvement with their patients.) Based on these three surveys, the rate of sexual misconduct by male psychiatrists is about 10 percent.

As a point of comparison, four self-report surveys of practicing psychologists carried out between 1977 and 1986 revealed that 4.8 to 12 percent of males and 0.8 to 3 percent of females had been sexually involved with current or former patients [21; 85; 139; 140].

How Common Is Sexual Misconduct by Psychiatry Residents? To my knowledge, there has been only one survey of sexual misconduct by psychiatry residents. In that study, Nanette Gartrell and her colleagues sent a self-report questionnaire to all 1,113 PGY-4 residents listed in the 1986 American Medical Association Physician Masterfile [57]. Of the 1,087 questionnaires that were delivered, 548 (50.4%) were returned, though not all respondents answered every question. Overall, 72.1 percent of the residents (85.7% of the males and 52.0% of the females) acknowledged having been sexually attracted to one or more patients. Most of these residents (78.3%) discussed their attraction with their supervisors—a discussion that was more likely if the resident had been in psychotherapy.

Five of 539 residents (0.9%) admitted to sexual involvement with patients. In two cases (a single heterosexual male and a married heterosexual male), the misconduct occurred in the PGY-4 year; in one case (a separated or divorced heterosexual female), it occurred in the PGY-1 year; in one case (a single homosexual male), it occurred during a medical student clerkship on psychiatry; and in one case (a married heterosexual male),

Table 3. Surveys of Sexual Misconduct by Practicing Psychiatrists

Authors; Publication Date	*Number and Source of Potential Respondents*	*Response Rate (%)*	*Rate of Sexual Involvement for Males (%)*	*Rate of Sexual Involvement for Females (%)*
Kardener et al. 1973 [92]	200 males randomly selected from county medical society	57	10	—
Gartrell et al. 1986 [56]	5,574 psychiatrists selected by every fifth name from AMA Physician Masterfile	26	7.1	3.1
Leggett 1994 [107]	506 Fellows of the RANZCP selected by every third name from Australian Fellows List	68	9.3	1.4

Abbreviations: AMA = American Medical Association; RANZCP = Royal Australian and New Zealand College of Psychiatrists

the timing was not specified. The rate of sexual involvement acknowledged by residents was considerably lower than that reported by practicing psychiatrists—almost certainly because the residents had less exposure to patients than their seniors had. In recent years psychiatry residency programs have given more attention to preventing sexual misconduct [63; 64; 145; 177], but it remains for future surveys to discover whether such efforts have been effective.

Is Sexual Involvement with Former Patients Sexual Misconduct? Some of the surveys listed in tables 2 and 3 asked physicians (including psychiatrists) whether they approved or disapproved of sexual involvement with patients. Although most physicians condemned such behavior with current patients, fewer believed it was inappropriate with former patients. In addition to those surveys, there have been two reports that have focused on the subject in greater detail. The first, by John Coverdale and his colleagues [31], surveyed 500 obstetrician-gynecologists, 500 ophthalmologists, 250 internists, and 250 family practitioners. The names of these physicians were randomly selected from the American Medical Association Physician Masterfile, and the sample was limited to physicians under fifty years of age. Of the 1,500 questionnaires sent out, 777 were returned, for an overall response rate of 53.7 percent. Questionnaires were completed by 257 obstetrician-gynecologists (51.4%), 259 ophthalmologists (51.8%), 127 internists (50.8%), and 134 family practitioners (53.6%). Although both male and female physicians were surveyed, the findings were not analyzed by the sex of the respondent.

The investigators asked whether certain behaviors were *usually, sometimes,* or *never appropriate* at several stages of the doctor-patient relationship, or whether the respondent had *no opinion* on the matter. Some of the results of this survey are summarized in table 4. I find them disturbing because so many physicians thought that sexual involvement—or behavior that could lead to it—was acceptable conduct with current or former patients.

The second report to focus on physicians' attitudes about sexual involvement with patients dealt exclusively with psychiatrists. This report, by Judith Herman and her colleagues [80], was part of the survey summarized in table 3 with Nanette Gartrell as the first author. As noted in that table, the investigators sent a questionnaire to 5,574 psychiatrists who were selected by taking every fifth name from the American Medical Association Physician Masterfile. Completed questionnaires were returned by 1,423 psychiatrists, for a response rate of 26 percent.

Table 4. Physicians' Approval of Certain Behaviors with Current or Former Patients

Behavior	*Physician Groups* Who Thought Behavior Was Sometimes or Usually Appropriate (%)*
During consultation	
Arranging to meet for lunch	31.7–46.3
Kissing	13.4–21.8
Sexual contact	0.0–0.8
While patient in treatment	
Meeting for lunch	47.1–56.4
Kissing	19.7–31.3
Sexual contact	3.2–12.5
After patient left treatment	
Meeting for lunch	73.9–82.8
Kissing	58.3–71.5
Sexual contact	47.0–59.1

Source: Modified with permission from John Coverdale et al., "National Survey on Physicians' Attitudes toward Social and Sexual Contact with Patients," *Southern Medical Journal* 87, no. 11 (1994): 1067–71.
*Groups consisted of 257 obstetrician-gynecologists, 259 ophthalmologists, 127 internists, and 134 family practitioners.

In the survey, sexual contact was defined as "contact which [is] intended to arouse or satisfy sexual desire in the patient, therapist, or both" [56, p. 1127]. Despite the clarity of this definition, some of the findings reported by Herman and her colleagues are presented in a contradictory way. On the one hand, the investigators note that 98 percent of the psychiatrists surveyed believed that sexual contact was always inappropriate during consultations or while the patient was in treatment. On the other hand, they note that 11 percent of the respondents believed that kissing a patient could be appropriate in some circumstances and that "less than 5% believed that fondling, sitting on a lap, disrobing, or genital contact is appropriate under any circumstances" [80, p. 165]. Although these two sets of findings seem difficult to reconcile, it is clear that the great majority of respondents disapproved of sexual contact with patients who were in treatment.

Herman and her colleagues also found that the majority of psychiatrists surveyed disapproved of sexual contact with patients who had left treatment: 64.6 percent thought that it was inappropriate, 26.9 percent thought that it could sometimes be appropriate, and 8.5 percent had no opinion on the matter. As with the physicians in other specialties surveyed by Coverdale and his colleagues, there was less censure of sexual contact with former patients than there was of such contact with current patients, but, across the board, psychiatrists were more disapproving of sexual involvement at any stage in the doctor-patient relationship than were nonpsychiatric physicians.

Even though more psychiatrists regarded sexual involvement with former patients as sexual misconduct than other physicians did, I take little comfort from the thought that a sizable number of my colleagues could find such behavior acceptable. For me, the most important thing is not that the psychiatrist and the patient are both adults, or that true love can happen at any time, or that the patient might have an acute problem that can be quickly and permanently resolved—for me, the most important thing is what it means to be a psychiatrist.

I understand that psychiatrists sometimes do things that, in the psychiatric context, are roughly equivalent to an ophthalmologist's removing a cinder from a patient's eye. Thus, a psychiatrist might do a single consultation on a surgical patient who has a postoperative delirium. In such cases, you could say that there is no professional relationship to speak of, so that if the psychiatrist subsequently met the patient they could ethically establish any type of nonprofessional relationship they wanted. The contrast between this situation and doing psychodynamic psychotherapy with a narcissistic patient for an hour a week, month after month, in which the most intimate details of the patient's life are discussed is clear. But what if the psychiatrist assessed the mood of a patient with major depression twice in two weeks while that patient's psychiatrist was on vacation, or saw a bereaved patient for four sessions to discuss the latter's ambivalent feelings about a deceased parent, or did eight sessions of cognitive-behavioral therapy with a phobic patient, or did three months of weekly supportive psychotherapy with a demoralized patient immediately after the latter's divorce? Would it be ethical for the psychiatrist to become sexually involved with any of these patients after the treatment ended? How would the psychiatrist know whether or not the former patient's participation in the sexual relationship was motivated by a lingering transference reaction? Would it make a difference if the psychiatrist did not believe in the concept of transference [53; 122]? Would a sexual relationship be appropriate with a 20-year-old former patient? With an 18-year-old one? Should it make any difference if the psychiatrist and the former patient live in a small town (where the psychiatrist might be the only one in practice) or in a large city? And what length of time would be needed to decide that the professional relationship—and therefore the patient's vulnerability to exploitation—was well and truly over? Is three months long enough? A year [7; 8]?

To translate all of the issues raised by such questions into a guide for ethical behavior would need a decision-tree of bewildering complexity (e.g., "If the former patient is 18 years of age or older but still living with his or her parents, and if the treatment occurred on a weekly basis and lasted between three and six months, then a sexual relationship could be established after an interval of 9 months, unless the former patient has moved back home after a divorce, in which case the interval must be 12 months"). And even if such an algorithm could be agreed upon by the nation's psychiatrists or their representatives in professional organizations, state laws would be—as they now are—quite different from one another in deciding what constitutes criminal behavior when psychotherapists have sexual relations with patients.

My major disagreement with an "algorithmic" approach to sexual misconduct is more fundamental than that it would be unwieldy and unworkable. In my view, the most important problem is that it would bury under a mountain of petty distinctions the question of what it means to be a psychiatrist. In the matter of treating patients, psychiatrists should be more concerned with their responsibilities than their rights. The best way for all psychiatrists to meet their responsibility to protect patients from exploitation is to hold that, once a person becomes a patient, that individual loses *forever* the potential to become certain other things—an intimate friend, a lover, a spouse, an adopted child, an employee, a business partner. There are many other people who can fill these roles in our lives, and we should turn to *them* for confiding, romantic, and commercial relationships. We expect that patients will trust us, and we must make it clear that they can. In my opinion, sexual involvement with former patients *is* sexual misconduct and I therefore support the position of the American Psychiatric Association: "Sexual activity with a current or former patient is unethical" [6, p. 5].

What to Do If the Patient Takes the Initiative. It can be very unsettling when patients communicate by dress, speech, or behavior that they want you to cross the boundary of the psychotherapeutic relationship. If it seems that the patient is sending a message indirectly, it is always possible that you have misinterpreted an innocent phenomenon. If you ignore it and wait to see if it occurs again, you can minimize the risk of such a mistake. Even if your interpretation is correct, ignoring it allows the patient to save face if he or she has misjudged you and permits you to decide whether, with this patient at this time in this type of psychotherapy, you want to pursue the matter in subsequent sessions or finesse it—assuming the message is never sent again.

The odds may be greater that something in the patient's dress, speech, or behavior is an invitation for you to leave the psychiatrist's role if it represents a change from the patient's baseline. A patient who has worn transparent blouses or unbuttoned shirts from the very first session may dress that way every day, and even though the patient is sending a message (and one that may eventually become a topic for discussion in psychotherapy), it is not necessarily an invitation for you to abandon the role of psychiatrist. When that something in the patient's dress is new, however, and you are sure that it does not reflect the beginning of a hypomanic episode or a state of intoxication, you should ask about it if the phenomenon is repeated. Your inquiry will be less awkward if it is introduced with a transition from something the patient has said (e.g., "On the subject of work, I noticed that, both last week and today, you wore a transparent blouse/unbuttoned shirt. Were you trying to send a message to a co-worker—or to someone else?"). In the discussion that follows, you may learn that the change in the patient's dress was provoked by a slighting remark from a friend and that the patient now wants to prove that he or she is attractive despite what the friend thinks. In such cases, the patient's change in dress is not intended specifically for you, and it need not lead to a discussion of what is appropriate in the psychotherapeutic relationship. When the change *is* intended specifically for you, it may not have an erotic goal (e.g., "You always seem so cool and distant. I just wanted to see if you were a human being—if you'd react.") or it may, indeed, have such a goal (e.g., "Well, I was hoping that you'd notice me as a man/woman rather than just a patient. And to tell the truth, I think you're very attractive."). In either of the latter two cases, you should review the ground rules for a psychotherapeutic relationship and decide with the patient whether he or she is committed to following them.

The same general approach can be adopted if the patient seems to be sending an indirect message through speech (e.g., calling you by your first name) or behavior (e.g., touching your arm as you open the door after the session). Here, it is possible that the patient is not inviting you to cross the boundary of the psychotherapeutic relationship but has merely spoken or acted spontaneously out of friendly, grateful, or affectionate feelings. When patients who make such gestures respect the boundaries of the relationship, they may become embarrassed or apologize for their unwarranted familiarity, and the incident is never repeated. Of course, patients who *are* indirectly inviting a different kind of relationship can also apologize (to permit a graceful retreat if rebuffed), but—all things considered—it might be better to reserve a discussion about the respective roles of psychiatrist and patient until the speech or behavior occurs a second time.

When the patient sends a direct message, through speech or action, that he or she wants to have physical contact with you or wants you to be a friend or a lover, your response should be equally direct. Spoken invitations can be introduced in a variety of ways:

- "This relationship is so lopsided—you know everything about me and I don't know anything about you. I want to get to know you—the *real* you."
- "I think you'd understand me a lot better if we spent some time together out of the office."
- "I feel so lonely. Nobody cares about me. You say you care about me, but you don't show it."

Statements such as these should prompt a review of the psychotherapeutic relationship and a discussion of why the patient's other relationships are not providing what he or she wants from you.

Although it is always important to document the significant events and themes of each session in your notes, it is especially important to record, verbatim, a patient's invitation for you to cross the psychotherapeutic boundary and how you responded to it. You should do this immediately following the session in order to make it as accurate as possible—something that may be of great help if a disappointed patient retaliates by falsely accusing you of a sexual impropriety [14; 70; 158].

Careful documentation is, if anything, even more important when the patient's invitation is enacted rather than spoken. The medicolegal situation today is little different from that in 1993, when Thomas Gutheil and Glen Gabbard cautioned:

From the viewpoint of current risk-management principles, a handshake is about the limit of social physical contact at this time. Of course, a patient who attempts a hug in the last session after 7 years of intense, intensive, and successful therapy should probably not be hurled across the room. However, most hugs from patients should be discouraged in tactful, gentle ways by words, body language, positioning, and so forth. Patients who deliberately or provocatively throw their arms around the therapist despite repeated efforts at discouragement should be stopped. An appropriate response is to step back, catch both wrists in your hands, cross the patient's wrists in front of you, so that the crossed arms form a barrier between bodies, and say firmly, "Therapy is a talking relationship; please sit down so we can discuss your not doing this any more." [71, p. 195]

It is the responsibility of the psychiatrist, not the patient, to prevent sexual involvement. When a patient takes the initiative in trying to change the nature of your relationship, you must discuss the matter with your psychotherapy supervisor and residency director before you see the patient again. These discussions will permit you to talk through an unsettling experience and get advice about what to do next. You should then note in the patient's chart that the discussions have taken place and the reasoning behind the approach you will use in upcoming sessions. If, despite your best efforts, the patient persists in speech or behavior that undermines the psychotherapeutic relationship, treatment should be terminated, with appropriate referral to another psychotherapist.

What to Do If You Want to Take the Initiative. You can—and will—have any number of unprofessional thoughts about your patients, but what you say and what you do should be entirely professional. Because the capacity of psychiatrists for self-deception and post-hoc justification is probably no different from that of anyone else, it is not surprising that some psychiatrists guilty of sexual misconduct have defended their actions as beneficial to their patients. In the survey conducted by Nanette Gartrell and her colleagues, for example, although 73 percent of the psychiatrists who had been sexually involved with patients reported that love or pleasure had been their motivation, 19 percent said that it had been "to enhance the patient's self-esteem and/or to provide a restitutive emotional experience for the patient" [56, p. 1128].

If you are lonely and want company, are troubled and want understanding, are wounded and want comfort, or are lustful and want release, you must never take advantage of a patient to obtain it. If there is no one else in your life to provide what you desire, never ask a patient to furnish it. If a patient's problems are sexual in nature, you must help resolve them as a psychiatrist, not as a surrogate. And even when you sense or know that a patient would readily comply with your wishes, you must never forget that the patient is just that—a patient.

If sexual thoughts about a patient interfere with your clinical reasoning, or if you worry that you might act on those thoughts, you must discuss your predicament with your psychotherapy supervisor and residency director. They should understand how such thoughts can develop in the context of psychotherapy [157], and they will help you decide how best to proceed. You may feel embarrassed to seek their advice, but the stakes for the patient, and for you, are very high.

The Use of First Names

There are issues other than sexual misconduct that should lead you to reflect on the boundaries of the psychotherapeutic relationship. One such issue is the use of first names. Although it is natural and appropriate to address children by their first names, I recommend that for adults you use titles (Mr., Mrs., Miss, etc.). I make this suggestion even though a survey of psychotherapists in Massachusetts revealed that most psychologists, many social workers, and some psychiatrists routinely called patients by their first names [159], and surveys of Australian and British psychiatric inpatients showed that the great majority of them wanted to be called by their first names [61; 147].

One reason I think it is better to address adult patients formally is to provide a measure of symmetry in what is a most asymmetrical relationship. Because patients will, almost without exception, address you by your title, you should address them by theirs. In so doing, you will demonstrate that you re-gard them as adults and, in the end, as equals.

Another reason to use titles when addressing adult patients is that none of them will be offended by it, whereas some (es-pecially those older than you) could feel demeaned if you call them by their first names. It would be quite difficult for many patients, especially at the start of a psychotherapeutic relation-ship, to protest and insist that you use their titles.

A final reason for addressing adult patients formally is to re-mind them of the professional nature of the relationship. When some patients (e.g., dependent or histrionic ones) are called by their first names, it may be easier for them to think of you as a kind of parent, friend, or potential lover who will magically solve their problems. A similar blurring of boundaries can occur if you try to obtain a measure of symmetry in the relationship by asking patients to call you by *your* first name. What you hope to convey by doing this and what the patient actually makes of it may be very different things.

Even when adult patients ask to be called by their first names, as they sometimes do on meeting you, I still think it is wise to use titles because at that point you have no idea why they are making the request. You can respond to a patient who asks to be called by his or her first name in a straightforward manner:

Psychiatrist: Hello, Mr. Franklin. I'm Alice Henry.

Patient: Hello, Doc.

Psychiatrist: Have a seat.

Patient: Thanks.

Psychiatrist: Did you sign in with the secretary?

Patient: Yes. She was very nice.

Psychiatrist: I'm glad to hear it. Well, Mr. Franklin, I know that Dr. Gomez referred you to the clinic because he thought you might be depressed, but I'd like you to tell me yourself what's been troubling you.

Patient: Sure, Doc, but you don't have to call me Mr. Franklin —you can just call me Charlie.

Psychiatrist: I appreciate the offer, Mr. Franklin, but in a pro-

fessional relationship like this, where you're going to call
me Doctor, I'd like to call you Mister. I hope that's all right.
Patient: Sure, Doc—it's just that most doctors call me Charlie.
Psychiatrist: Well, this doctor is going to call you Mr. Franklin.
Okay?
Patient: Okay.

Your Dress and Grooming

As a physician, you dress not only for yourself but also for your
role. Because your role is more specifically that of a resident
physician, your dress is determined, to a greater or lesser degree,
by the expectations of your program. Thus, for example, the
wearing of a white coat may be encouraged in one residency and
discouraged in another. Whatever the expectations of your program, your dress and grooming should not hamper your relationship with patients. It is one thing to wear a religious sym-
bol; it would be quite another to wear a tongue stud.

Surveys of general medical patients have revealed that, among
patients who express a preference about the dress of their physicians, most want them to look "professional" (i.e., to dress more,
rather than less, formally) [36; 116; 118]. I could find only two
surveys of patients' attitudes about the dress of psychiatrists: one
found that 49 British urban inpatients preferred more formal
attire [61]; the other found that 58 Australian rural outpatients
preferred less formal attire [142]. No general conclusion can be
drawn from these two small studies except perhaps that opinions can vary with locale.

The best way to make sure that your appearance does not im-
pede the psychotherapeutic relationship is to put yourself in
your patients' shoes and imagine what effect it might have on
them. Because patients in different places might have somewhat
different standards about what kind of dress and grooming are
appropriate for physicians, your appearance should approximate
local norms. If your dress and grooming differ greatly from
those norms, your patients may make assumptions about you
(e.g., that you lack respect for them, that you are not serious
about your work) which could be quite wrong.

Your Office

Because your office, like your dress and grooming, says something about you, you may wonder how its decor affects the psychotherapeutic relationship. Should the desk be positioned between you and the patient or against the wall? Should you display pictures of family members? Although psychiatrists now seem less concerned with such questions than they were a generation or two ago [96], it is still important to think about the layout and appearance of your office from a patient's point of view.

The matter is complicated to some extent by the fact that you are a resident, which means not only that you change offices several times a year but also that the offices you occupy have already been furnished and painted to someone else's taste and budget. Despite these constraints, you can still put your personal stamp on your surroundings.

Although the arrangement of furniture in an office (e.g., how close the chairs are to one another, where the desk is placed) would seem to have a measurable effect on the comfort levels of psychotherapists and patients, such relationships have been studied only in simulated or single-session interviews, not in actual, ongoing psychotherapy [59; 151]. Even without such studies, however, you know by now how a certain type of environment affects you, and in some cases you can tell—or guess—how it affects your patients. A paranoid patient, for example, may be more comfortable if he or she has unimpeded access to the door and is seated on the opposite side of the desk from you.

In the end, because you spend much more time in your office than any of your patients do, you should arrange and decorate it to suit your needs and preferences. It will make little difference to patients whether you have diplomas, Impressionist prints, or departmental schedules on the wall, but they might be disenchanted to see that you left a pile of clothes in the corner after a night on duty.

Self-Disclosure

I use the term *self-disclosure* here to refer to things that you reveal about yourself by what you say (e.g., that you play the piano,
that your parents divorced when you were nine) rather than
things you reveal about yourself by how you speak (e.g., that you
grew up in the South, that you are a stickler for grammar), how
you dress (e.g., that you like blue, that you are a Christian), or
how you decorate your office (e.g., that you are messy, that you
graduated from Ohio State).

You can disclose things about yourself because a patient asks
you to or because you decide to. Most patients want to know
more about their psychiatrists than can be deduced from posters
on the wall or photographs on the desk, but not much more.
They may ask you to reveal information that is, in a sense, public (e.g., where you went to medical school, when you will finish
your residency) or somewhat private (e.g., the ages of your children, whether you enjoyed your vacation), but they usually do
not ask you to reveal information that is truly private (e.g., the
state of your marriage, how much money you make), either because they know it is inappropriate to do so or because they have
no interest in such matters.

Many psychiatrists readily reveal public and somewhat private
information in response to a patient's request when they judge
the disclosure to be helpful or neutral in terms of the psychotherapeutic relationship. Those same psychiatrists, however,
usually refuse to reveal truly private information, not only because they believe it would erode the boundary of the psychotherapeutic relationship but also because they know it might
make it harder to discover the patient's motivation for asking.
One reason why a patient might ask about your most private life
is that he or she has fantasies about being your friend, or sib-
ling, or lover, and so wants to know more about you as a person
rather than as a psychiatrist. Another reason might be that the
patient fears that he or she will break down if the discussion
continues on its current line and asks a question to change the
subject. If, in the hope of making a therapeutic point or of

demonstrating your commitment to a symmetrical relationship, you disclose the private information the patient has requested, you may find that *your* life, rather than that of the patient, has become the focus of the session:

> *Patient:* We're always talking about problems with my marriage—what about your marriage? Don't you ever quarrel with your husband?
>
> *Psychiatrist:* Of course I do, every once in a while.
>
> *Patient:* Well, what do you quarrel about? I bet it's the same things—the kids, money, sex. Do you want sex every time he does?

You can deflect such questions and still preserve the opportunity to discover the patient's motivation for asking:

> *Patient:* We're always talking about problems with my marriage—what about your marriage? Don't you ever quarrel with your husband?
>
> *Psychiatrist:* What difference would it make if I did or I didn't?
>
> *Patient:* Well, if you did, maybe I wouldn't feel like I was the only one who couldn't make a man happy.
>
> *Psychiatrist:* Make a man happy?
>
> *Patient:* Isn't that what you're supposed to do? My mother didn't have a life of her own because she was supposed to make my father happy. I don't want to end up like her!

In addition to disclosing information at the request of patients, you can also disclose it without being asked. Such voluntary disclosures should not be taken lightly, for there is an important difference between saying what you think or feel as a psychiatrist and saying what you think or feel as a private individual. As a psychiatrist, you must convey certain thoughts and emotions to patients in order to help them change. Thus, it is perfectly appropriate to say that you are worried to hear that a patient has decided on a dangerous course of action or that you are happy to hear that a patient has achieved a long-sought goal.

The disclosure of these feelings keeps the focus on the patient and leads naturally to a further discussion of the patient's situation (e.g., "Now that you've got the job, do you anticipate any problems?").

There are a few circumstances in which psychiatrists, *as* psychiatrists, volunteer private information because such disclosures are common in those circumstances and are made to benefit patients. If, for example, you work in a substance abuse program because you were an alcoholic and want to help other alcoholics, you might reveal your own history to patients as evidence that you can understand their problem and as proof that someone can overcome an addiction. In making this disclosure, you would almost certainly be acting like other psychotherapists in the program who had been addicts themselves.

There are also a few circumstances in which psychiatrists, *as* psychiatrists, have a duty to volunteer private information because patients, *as* patients, have a right to know it. If, for example, you believe on religious grounds that abortion is murder, that women who have abortions are sinful, and that it is your responsibility to prevent abortions, you must disclose that information to patients considering abortions. Those patients have a right to know that your advice on the subject may be based on religious rather than clinical principles, and they should be asked if, under the circumstances, they wish to be treated elsewhere. Another example of voluntary disclosure of private information that patients have a right to know is that you have a sustained feeling about the patient (e.g., love, mistrust) that has compromised your professional judgment. If this occurs, the patient must be referred to another psychotherapist.

Voluntary disclosures of private information such as those illustrated above preserve the boundaries of the psychotherapeutic relationship. There are also, however, voluntary disclosures that violate those boundaries. It is, for example, inappropriate for psychiatrists to tell patients that they are sexually attracted to them, unless that is given as the reason for terminating treatment. Although it has been argued that such disclosures (e.g., "I think you should know I'm feeling sexually aroused right now. Are you aware that you've been acting seductively?") can be therapeutically useful, I believe that they are much more likely to have the opposite effect. Many patients would think it un-professional for a psychiatrist to reveal sexual feelings, while others would be threatened by the revelation or use it as the basis for fantasies or behaviors that distract them from their original goals in treatment. Psychiatrists who are excited by the possibility of sexual conquest, who long for sympathetic under-standing, or who are greedy for power over others may make dis-closures that gratify their own needs at the expense of those of their patients. Such actions exploit the psychotherapeutic rela-tionship to take advantage of people who have made themselves vulnerable in order to be helped. In my opinion, most inappro-priate self-disclosures are not made with predatory intent, but on the basis of therapeutic zeal or naïveté. Although it is always important to think twice before disclosing private information, psychiatrists should be especially reflective when their own re-lationships are failing, when they are ill, when their work no longer satisfies them, or when they are suffering financial diffi-culties [18; 180]. If you are in doubt whether or not to disclose pri-vate information or think you have done so inappropriately, you should discuss the matter with your psychotherapy supervisor.

Calls at Home

One of the things you and your patients must discuss at the start of treatment is how they can contact you in case of emergency. Depending on your personality, your current rotation, your liv-ing arrangements, among other factors, some of you will give patients your telephone or pager number; others of you will ask them to call the hospital's answering service or emergency room. And depending on your assessment of a given patient's personality and clinical state, you will set a higher or lower threshold for such contacts—a threshold that may vary over the course of treatment. Even though you and your patients agree on the indications for calling you at night or on weekends, some of them will do it less often than you think they should, while others will do it more often than you wish them to.

There are many reasons why patients might want to speak to you outside of scheduled psychotherapy sessions. It may be, for example, that they are suicidal and want to be stopped; that they feel overwhelmed and want support; that they are paralyzed by doubt and need advice; that they are angry with you and want to punish you by disrupting your life; that they are in love with you and want to hear your voice. If a patient calls repeatedly and appropriately in the midst of a crisis, you should consider scheduling the calls—something that will reassure the patient of your availability and spare you unexpected interruptions.

Whenever patients call you at home, there is a chance that they will speak to or hear your housemate, spouse, or children. Although this might lead the patient to ask for private information you would not have volunteered, you can often deal with the request in a matter-of-fact way. Thus, for example, if a patient phones you at home and asks if the person who answered was your spouse, you can simply say, "Yes" or "No, it was my sister" and direct the conversation back to the reason for the patient's call. If, in the psychotherapy session following that call, the patient wants to know the name of your spouse or sister, you can provide it (or not) and again redirect the conversation. Most patients understand the boundaries of the psychotherapeutic relationship and will be satisfied with a minimum of information. If patients request more information than you wish to disclose, you can remind them of the nature of the psychotherapeutic relationship (e.g., that it is an asymmetrical one) and again direct the conversation to the patient's situation.

Whenever a patient phones you at home and other people are present, you should take the call in a private setting, both to assure the patient that he or she has your full attention and to minimize the chance that the patient will draw erroneous conclusions about you from voices or sounds in the background. You might also reduce the chance of erroneous conclusions if the message on your telephone answering machine is reasonably dignified.

Chance Meetings

Although chance meetings between psychiatrists and patients are more likely in small towns than in large cities, you can bump into patients no matter where you live. When you encounter patients in a mall, at a movie, in a restaurant, or at a party, the situation can be awkward—both for the patients and for you. Your behavior in these circumstances is generally best guided by what the patients do. Some of them will not acknowledge you because they too want privacy, but in the next psychotherapy session they may mention that they saw you in such-and-such a place and ask who you were with. Other patients will greet you and exchange a few words. If you are alone when this occurs, there is usually no problem, but if you are with your spouse or a friend, it gets more complicated. The best thing to do when you have a companion is simply to introduce the parties by name, but not to disclose that the patient is a patient (e.g., "Frank, this is Barbara Saunders. Mrs. Saunders, this is my husband, Frank Chen."). Spouses often know the names of patients (e.g., because they have called you at home) or quickly learn that your manner of introducing patients identifies them as such. If you are with an inquisitive friend when you meet a patient and you wish to protect the patient's status, you can simply tell the friend that the patient is someone you know from the hospital. All of this is much easier, of course, if the patients decide to identify themselves as patients when you introduce them to your companion.

If you treat students or house officers at your medical school, chance meetings on campus are common but easily dealt with, for you and the patient can exchange greetings that reflect your roles in the institution, rather than your roles in psychotherapy. When you encounter such patients at parties, however, things can be quite awkward, for you and the patient will be constrained by your psychotherapeutic relationship at the same time that other partygoers may be encouraging you to hold forth or to unwind. If that occurs, you can change the subject or excuse yourself from the conversation—actions the patient may take as well. You and the patient can then discuss the encounter in the next psychotherapy session and decide how to deal with similar situations in the future. Treating colleagues—or the family members of colleagues—is a fact of life for many physicians. In such circumstances you may well be able to manage the dual role of distant colleague and psychiatrist, but you should never attempt to be the psychiatrist of a close colleague or a friend.

Accepting Gifts

Patients may offer you small gifts on holidays, after you have expressed an interest in their hobbies, when they are especially appreciative of your efforts on their behalf, and on completion of treatment. Such gifts should generally be accepted in the spirit in which they are offered, rather than made the focus of psychotherapeutic inquiry (e.g., "Perhaps you could tell me what you were thinking when you chose the candy?"). Most psychiatrists are probably much more reluctant to accept a gift certificate than, say, a box of homemade cookies, but they might accept the gift certificate if it has a personal quality. Thus, for example, if a patient offers you a gift certificate to a restaurant, he or she may say, "It's one of my favorite places. I hope you'll enjoy it, too." Patients rarely offer cash as a gift, which is fortunate because most psychiatrists would refuse it (e.g., "I appreciate the thought, but you already pay me for my services, so I'm afraid I can't accept it"). If a patient entreats you to take a cash gift after you have declined it, you can suggest that the patient give it to a worthy cause in your name.

There are, of course, situations in which a gift should be refused and the patient's reason for offering it should be explored. A patient may, for example, try to give you something session after session or press you to accept an expensive gift. Such behavior might express a vulnerability in the patient's personality (e.g., a tendency to curry favor with authority figures that later leads to self-loathing) or it might be an attempt on the patient's part to convert a professional relationship into a personal one.

4. Psychotherapy Supervision

Learning psychotherapy is like learning surgery: although you can read about it in articles and books, mastery comes with supervised experience. Because the process of acquiring experience is a long one, it is not surprising that some beginning residents embrace a "school" of psychotherapy in hopes that knowledge of its theories and techniques will confer mastery more quickly. These hopes may be encouraged by supervisors who believe that their effectiveness as psychotherapists is derived from the teachings of the school to which they belong. This is an understandable opinion, but one that may well be incorrect, for (as noted in chapter 3) there is evidence to suggest that the relationship between the psychotherapist and the patient is a more important determinant of outcome than the theories or techniques the psychotherapist employs. Although I have discussed some aspects of psychotherapeutic theory in connection with life-story reasoning and the psychotherapeutic relationship, I return to the subject of theory here in order to examine its influence on beginning residents and their supervisors.

Psychotherapeutic Theories: Positives and Negatives

Psychotherapeutic theories can help beginners by closing gaps in a patient's life story. If, for example, you are puzzled by a female patient's domineering behavior toward the men in her life despite their evident high regard for her as a daughter, a sister, a wife, and a colleague, your familiarity with a variety of psychotherapeutic theories would allow you to consider themes that could account for the paradox. One such theme, Alfred Adler's concept of "masculine protest" [1, pp. 87–88], might permit you to connect the patient's behavior with her belief that, because it is still a male-dominated world, the only way she can overcome her feelings of inferiority is to act as she thinks a man would act—assertively. This meaningful connection would bring coherence to the patient's life story and thereby contribute to its "narrative truth" (see chapter 1). Once you can tell a coherent story, you feel more confident that you are on the right track.

Another way—albeit a dangerous one—in which psychotherapeutic theories can increase the confidence of beginners was suggested by Jerome Frank:

> A therapist can succeed only if he has some conviction that what he is doing makes sense and that he is competent to do it. He gains this feeling first of all from his therapeutic successes, which, often erroneously, he regards as evidence for the validity of his theory. That is, a patient's improvement may actually have resulted from aspects of the therapeutic situation that escape the therapist's formulations and even his notice, such as the rebirth of hope. The success rate of most psychotherapists, however, is scarcely large enough to sustain their self-confidence. It is a rare therapist who has not experienced periods of discouragement and self-doubt. At such moments . . . adherence to a doctrine may be a major source of emotional support, and the most supportive, hence the most seductive, theories explain away the therapist's failures while letting him take credit for his successes. That is, successes are proof of the theory's validity while failures cannot shake it. [43, pp. 147–48]

Beginners who embrace a psychotherapeutic theory that purports to explain all emotional distress in terms of a few simple ideas become very confident, and very limited, psychotherapists. Such beginners know in advance why patients are suffering and tell the same life story for all of them. When this happens, patients disappear as individuals and become mere exemplars of the story's main theme, whether of castration anxiety, birth trauma, the persona and the anima, or repressed sexual abuse. Hilde Bruch warned beginners of this danger as it applies to psychoanalysis, but her point is valid for all psychotherapeutic theories:

Learning specific theories and therapeutic techniques, psychoanalytic or otherwise, may be stimulating and give the reassurance that one has been let in on some secret knowledge; to some it may be of help in organizing observations. But the beginner needs to realize that this knowledge does not give him any help when he sits down with a patient. It does not tell you what to say to a patient or what to listen for, and it may even make you focus on something which, according to the theory, should be there and thus stand in the way of hearing what the patient is trying to say. . . .

On the surface it may not seem to matter whether one refers to Mr. X as doing or saying this or that, or whether one speaks of his having strong or weak ego functions. The telling difference is that in one image the patient is conceived of as a person who is living his own life, though inefficiently and beset with all kinds of problems; in the other, the person is conceived of as a container that houses the various "mechanisms" or "ego functions" which determine what he does. [23, p. 85]

One of the best psychotherapy supervisors I had as a resident was a very experienced psychoanalyst who shared Bruch's opinion about the place of theory in the education of beginners. Whenever I asked him whether a patient's behavior represented, say, "identification with the aggressor," he would gently turn aside the question and ask me how I understood the behavior in terms of the patient's personality, family relationships, and social circumstances. He was very interested in *exactly* what she said and did, and his interpretations and predictions were always grounded in the particulars of the case, rather than in theoretical constructs. I had no doubt that he knew psychoanalytic theory, but what he was teaching me was the product of twenty-five years of experience as a psychotherapist.

Psychotherapeutic Theories and Clinical Experience

In 1950, Fred Fiedler published three small studies examining the relative importance of psychotherapeutic theories and clinical experience in determining the relationship psychotherapists attempt to create with their patients. In the first two studies [41], he found that psychologists and psychiatrists from a variety of backgrounds (psychoanalytic, Rogerian, Adlerian, eclectic) were in general agreement about statements most characteristic of an ideal psychotherapeutic relationship (e.g., "An empathic relationship"; "Therapist sticks closely to the patient's problems"; "The patient assumes an active role") and statements least characteristic of such a relationship (e.g., "An impersonal, cold relationship"; "The therapist curries favor with the patient"; "The therapist tries to impress the patient with his skill or knowledge"). He also found that well-educated people with no training as psychotherapists ranked a series of 75 statements about the psychotherapeutic relationship in the same way that psychologists and psychiatrists did. Fiedler concluded that the participants' notion of an ideal psychotherapeutic relationship was not derived from theories but from what they regarded as good interpersonal relationships in general.

In the third study [40], Fiedler used the same 75 statements about the psychotherapeutic relationship to assess actual psychotherapy sessions. He asked three psychotherapists (one each from psychoanalytic, Rogerian, and eclectic orientations) and one lay person to listen to recorded excerpts of psychotherapy sessions conducted by 10 different psychotherapists. Among the 10 were two expert psychoanalysts, two novice psychoanalysts, two expert Rogerian therapists, two novice Rogerian therapists, one expert Adlerian therapist, and one novice Adlerian therapist. After listening to each excerpt, the judges ranked the 75 statements according to whether they were the most, or the least, characteristic of the session from which the excerpt was taken. Whereas Fiedler's earlier studies had described the qualities of an ideal psychotherapeutic relationship, this study assessed the qualities of actual relationships. His analysis of the judges' ratings led Fiedler to the following conclusions:

(1) Expert psychotherapists of any of the three schools create a relationship more closely approximating the Ideal Thera-

peutic Relationship than relationships created by non-experts.

(2) The therapeutic relationship created by experts of one school resembles more closely that created by experts of other schools than it resembles relationships created by nonexperts within the same school.

(3) The most important dimension (of those measured) which differentiates experts from nonexperts is related to the therapist's ability to understand, to communicate with, and to maintain rapport with the patient. [p. 444]

These three studies suggest that experience, more than theory, determines the type of relationship expert psychotherapists attempt to establish with their patients. If this is true, and if the relationship is crucial to the success or failure of treatment, then what you want most from your psychotherapy supervisors is not their theoretical knowledge but their clinical wisdom.

The Focus of Supervision

At various times during the course of psychotherapy supervision, your supervisor will ask you to focus on the patient, on your relationship with the patient, or on yourself [68]. When you present a new patient to a supervisor, the focus is naturally on the patient, for the supervisor's primary responsibility is to help you make an accurate diagnosis, design an appropriate plan of treatment, and further the patient's progress. When that progress is slow or erratic, your supervisor may ask you to focus on your relationship with the patient, so that rather than discussing phenomena such as the patient's symptoms or changing life circumstances, you and the supervisor discuss phenomena such as the vicissitudes of the therapeutic alliance and the possibility that the patient is having a transference reaction. Sometimes when the patient is not doing well, but more often when you become demoralized or anxious about the progress of treatment, your supervisor may ask you to focus on yourself. As

I noted in chapter 2, your supervisor should be able to help you minimize your trait-related problems as they affect your care of patients without making you a patient yourself. Thus, for example, if you become discouraged because a difficult patient has shown little improvement, your supervisor may not only reassure you that the patient's personality is the main obstacle to progress but also speculate whether you might be distressed, in part, because you tend to be self-doubting and self-critical. You might have mentioned those traits yourself when discussing a different case, or your supervisor might have noticed them as he or she has gotten to know you over time. If you think the supervisor is correct, the two of you can talk about ways in which you can emphasize the benefits of those characteristics and diminish their burdens. If you think the supervisor is wrong, you should say so, and the two of you can shift your focus back to the patient or to your relationship with the patient.

In days gone by, it was more common for psychotherapy supervisors to focus on the supervisee, even at the beginning of supervision. This practice was based on the assumption, discussed in chapter 2, that psychiatrists need psychotherapy to be competent psychotherapists. Although many supervisors who made this assumption also believed that they could not—and should not—be both a teacher and a psychotherapist for their supervisees, they also believed that self-awareness was important for psychotherapists and that it was their responsibility to help their students become more self-aware. For these supervisors, the best setting in which to demonstrate the need for self-awareness was the supervisor-supervisee relationship, for both parties in that relationship could function as participant-observers. It was, I believe, such reasoning that led to an awkward exchange between one of my supervisors and me during our first meeting. I had just given what I thought was a thorough presentation of a complicated case and I was eager for his guidance. He began not by asking me for more information about the patient, nor by asking me to expand on my diagnostic formulation, nor by asking me to propose a plan of treatment—instead, he began by asking me why I had not told him the name of a psychiatrist who had briefly treated the patient the year before. When I responded that the treatment had lasted only a few sessions, that it had not gone well, and that I was not sure whether he knew the psychiatrist, who may have been unfairly criticized, he said, "Well, Phillip, the fact that you didn't tell me the psychiatrist's name says something about what you think of me." I was so nonplussed by his statement that I could only blurt out: "Um. . . . If you want me to tell you what I think of you, I'll tell you. Do you want me to tell you what I think of you?" It was now his turn to be dumbfounded (because, I believe, no resident had ever spoken to him like that before), and he only harrumphed and directed the conversation back to the patient.

If a psychotherapy supervisor insists on discussing your personality or your personal life when there seems no reason to do so, you should ask your residency director for a different supervisor, just as you should if a supervisor repeatedly misses sessions, usually falls asleep, or makes sexual advances. Fortunately, such behaviors are rare. In every residency program there should be wise, kind, experienced psychotherapy supervisors who will help you learn a difficult craft.

Fear of Criticism: A Potential Obstacle to Supervision

Most beginning residents are eager to have psychotherapy supervision, but that eagerness is often tempered by fear of criticism. As Stanley Greben has noted:

> The greatest pleasure for talented and interested residents is the regular opportunity to discuss psychotherapy cases with an experienced clinician and teacher. In the first year of residency, residents are intimidated by the expectation that they would engage in psychotherapy with any patient. Whatever little reading they have done on the subject has given them vague ideas of how to proceed, but no degree of confidence that they can adequately fill the role of psychotherapist. They are afraid that they may not be able to say anything useful

and, even more, that they may say something wrong or damaging to the patient. . . . The psychotherapy hours seem hopelessly complicated, and they are all too aware that as careful a record as they make of the proceedings, in order to be able to report fairly to their supervisor, that record will be a pallid shadow of what has actually taken place in therapy.

Residents come to their early meetings with a new supervisor with some apprehension. Will they be chided or humiliated? Will they be exposed as too supportive or laissez-faire? Will their ignorance of psychoanalysis or psychodynamic psychiatry be woefully evident? [66, pp. 307–8]

To avoid criticism and shame, residents sometimes "edit" their reports of psychotherapy sessions [74]. This practice, while understandable, deprives both the patient and the resident of the supervisor's best advice. The potential for omitting or fabricating material in order to avoid criticism is greatest when written notes are used as the basis for supervision, but it is also possible to edit audiotapes and videotapes—if not to create an impression of having done something, at least to create an impression of not having done something. Deception is impossible, of course, when the supervisor observes the session through a one-way mirror or acts as co-therapist in group psychotherapy, but in most residency programs direct supervision is the exception, not the rule. Direct supervision demands even more time from busy supervisors, and residents usually do not press for it, perhaps because it is the supervisory setting in which they have the least privacy and therefore the least chance of saving face [16].

Being supervised in any fashion is uncomfortable for residents who mistake a supervisor's observations and conjectures for criticisms. If you have this tendency, you might want to tell your supervisor about it so that he or she can appropriately label remarks. Of course, there *are* hypercritical supervisors, and if you feel that you have one, you should discuss your predicament with your residency director. In the end, it is up to the supervisor to provide an environment conducive to learning and to determine what help you need most; in the end, it is up to you to be forthright.

Other Potential Obstacles to Supervision

The Attitude That Psychotherapy Is Not for Psychiatrists

The attitude that psychotherapy is not for psychiatrists has been promoted, in part, by psychiatrists themselves. There have been three elements in the growth of this opinion. First, it became clear that certain schools of psychotherapy had failed in their claims to understand the cause of psychiatric disorders and to offer effective treatments for those conditions. Second, the increasing pace of discovery in neuroscience and related fields has given us medications that can help patients in ways that psychotherapy never could. Here, for example, I mean not only that neuroleptics are useful for "psychotic" phenomena such as hallucinations and delusions but also that selective serotonin reuptake inhibitors are useful for "neurotic" phenomena such as obsessions and panic attacks. Finally, as psychiatry has become more like other medical specialties in its use of the scientific method, some psychiatrists have adopted a narrow and mistaken view of what they, as physicians, should be doing. This view depends on the following syllogism:

Major Premise: Physicians treat diseases.

Minor Premise: Psychiatrists are physicians.

Conclusion: If the patient's complaints are due not to a disease (of the brain) but to problems in living, then the treatment of those complaints is a matter not for psychiatrists, but for psychologists, social workers, nurses, and other counselors.

The fundamental problem with such reasoning is, of course, in the major premise, for physicians treat patients, not diseases. Many physicians care for patients who are troubled rather than diseased, and some of those physicians are excellent psychotherapists, within the constraints of their practice.

To the extent that academic psychiatrists—especially directors of departments and residency programs—believe that psychotherapy is a thing of the past, a second-rate treatment, to that extent they will devalue the place of psychotherapy supervision in your education. For residency programs to be accredited, they must provide a certain amount of supervision, but some faculty members in programs that seek to produce "brain doctors" may look down on residents who are interested in psychotherapy, just as some faculty members in programs that sought to produce "mind doctors" once looked down on residents who were interested in neuroscience.

Another reason for the attitude that psychotherapy is not for psychiatrists is the change in medical practice brought about by managed care. As Paul Summergrad and his colleagues noted: "The major managed-care companies, for-profit and working in the private sector, do not permit residents to treat their members. Although a master's-prepared clinician is considered 'qualified,' even a senior psychiatric resident with an outstanding record from a nationally regarded institution and with much more training is considered inadequate" [171, p. 256]. One result of such policies is that fewer cases—especially those suitable for long-term psychotherapy—are available for supervision. Another result is that graduating psychiatrists increasingly believe that psychotherapy not only can be done by psychologists, social workers, nurses, and other counselors, but that it *should* be done by them. If this view becomes more widespread, the pool of psychiatrists qualified to be psychotherapy supervisors will soon diminish. (The advent of managed care has, of course, affected residency education in areas other than psychotherapy supervision [20; 83; 187].)

Prejudice, Ignorance, or Insensitivity by the Supervisor or the Resident

The race, culture, gender, or sexual orientation of the resident or supervisor can become an obstacle to supervision if either party in the relationship is prejudiced, ignorant, or insensitive about such matters. Relatively little has been written about this topic, perhaps because it is so awkward to study. It would be re-assuring to believe that people who are interested in psychiatry tend to be tolerant of others in general and that psychiatrists tend to be tolerant of one another because so many of us belong to minority groups, but such beliefs have not been validated. Indeed, it is possible that diversity among psychiatrists provides more opportunity for prejudice, ignorance, and insensitivity than would exist if we were a more homogeneous group.

The one thing that cannot be doubted in all of this is that psychiatry residents are a fairly varied lot. Their diversity is reflected in the American Psychiatric Association's 2001–2002 Resident Census, which had an 83.2 percent response rate (5,766 residents) from 493 accredited residencies and fellowships [4]. That survey revealed, for example, that male and female residents were equally common, and that 38.6 percent of residents were international medical graduates. Racial identification was not provided by 7.9 percent of the respondents, but 58.0 percent identified themselves white, 24.6 percent as Asian, 6.7 percent as Black/African American, 0.4 percent as Native Hawaiian/Other Pacific Islander, 0.3 percent as American Indian/Alaska Native, and 2.1 percent as Other. Residents of Hispanic ethnicity reported a variety of racial identifications and constituted 3.3 percent of the total. The APA census did not assess sexual orientation, but a survey of all Canadian psychiatry residents with a response rate of 58.7 percent revealed that 94.3 percent of the respondents described themselves as heterosexual, 4.1 percent as homosexual, and 1.6 percent as bisexual [25].

These American and Canadian surveys provide a context for considering how prejudice, ignorance, and insensitivity about matters of race, culture, gender, or sexual orientation might interfere with psychotherapy supervision. In one of the few papers on this general topic in the last decade, Carol Nadelson and her colleagues discussed the influence of gender and sexual orientation on the supervisory process [129]. They noted, for example, that communication may be distorted when supervisors assume that residents are heterosexual. If such an assumption is evident to homosexual residents, some of them may disguise their sexual orientation or refuse to present homosexual patients for supervision. Because Nadelson and her colleagues were interested in a resident perspective on how issues of gender and sexual orientation affect the supervisory process, one of the paper's authors, Keith Ablow, conducted an informal survey of residents in the Boston area. The survey revealed, among other things, that heterosexual residents disapproved of homosexuality in supervisors of either sex, and that homosexual residents tended to prefer homosexual supervisors.

Ronald Ruskin also addressed the ways in which prejudice, ignorance, and insensitivity might interfere with psychotherapy supervision, though his focus was on race and culture rather than on gender and sexual orientation:

> The supervisee from another culture may feel misunderstood, marginalized, responded to in an indifferent or prejudicial manner, and unable to express his or her particular perspectives. Cultural divergences may make the supervisee more vigilant and anxious about the supervisor's capacity to attend to and critically evaluate the supervisee's experience and performance. When the supervisee comes from a different country, speaks a different mother tongue, is a member of a racial or ethnic minority, and/or is of a different religion from the dominant culture supervisor, the capacity to identify with the supervisor may be made more difficult than with a colleague who shares similar or convergent cultural determinants. [149, pp. 59–60]

If you find that one of your supervisors is prejudiced, ignorant, or insensitive about you or your patients and you do not want to raise the issue with the supervisor in question, you should bring the matter to the attention of your residency director. If you are correct about the supervisor, the odds are that he or she will apologize and try to do better; if you are wrong— and acknowledge it—the supervisor's self-esteem and reputation should be restored.

It is possible, of course, that *you* may be prejudiced, ignorant, or insensitive, and that your criticisms of a supervisor have less to do with that individual's skills as a teacher or clinician than with his or her race, culture, gender, or sexual orientation. If you realize you have such a problem, you are already on the road to correcting it. Depending on what you have said or how you have acted, an apology to the supervisor may or may not be appropriate. In any event, you will have learned something important about yourself.

An Impaired Supervisor

Psychiatrists are no less vulnerable to psychiatric disorders than other people are, and some psychiatrists are better at preaching the value of treatment than they are at accepting it. If your psychotherapy supervisor becomes impaired by a medical or surgical condition, he or she will almost certainly tell you about it and schedule a break in supervision or ask your residency director to provide a substitute. If, however, the impairment is due to a psychiatric disorder that distorts the supervisor's judgment, he or she may continue treating patients and supervising residents. If your supervisor is manic, profoundly depressed, very anxious, or repeatedly intoxicated, it will be obvious—and upsetting—to you. For the sake of your patients, the supervisor's patients, the supervisor, and the integrity of the residency program, you must tell your residency director what you have observed. If the impairing disorder is more subtle in its manifestations or if the supervisor tries to conceal it by missing sessions, it may take some time until you realize that he or she may be ill. In that case you will probably find it more awkward to speak to your residency director, but you should do so nonetheless. If you try to protect an impaired supervisor, you may only make matters worse.

I was able to find only two studies on the impact of impaired supervisors on residents. The first study, conducted by Kasia Kozlowska and her colleagues in Australia [100; 101], assessed many aspects of residents' experiences with patients, teachers, and peers. In 1994, the investigators sent a self-report questionnaire to all 137 house officers in New South Wales who had

completed at least one year of training and to all 95 consultants
(the equivalent of board-certified psychiatrists) in New South
Wales who had achieved specialist status within the previous five
years. Of the 232 questionnaires distributed, 178 (76.7%) were
completed and returned: 110 of them from trainees (completion
rate: 80.3%) and 68 from consultants (completion rate: 71.6%).

The investigators were particularly interested in the frequency
of adverse experiences for trainees and specifically inquired
about 20 potentially distressing situations, including that of
being supervised by a consultant whose psychiatric disorder
made the work environment unpleasant. Forty-five of the respondents (25.3%) endorsed having had such a supervisor, and
28 of them wrote comments on the question. These comments
included the trainee's diagnostic impression of the disorder impairing the supervisor. Although the investigators did not list all
of these diagnoses, they noted that in seven cases it was alcohol
abuse; in another seven, depression; in six, mania; in four, personality disorder; and in one, "psychosis." Three of the respondents said that the impaired supervisor's colleagues did not intervene in the situation.

In the second study on the impact of impaired supervisors on
residents, Karine Igartua sent a self-report questionnaire to all
600 psychiatry residents enrolled in Canadian programs in the
1996–1997 academic year [90]. The questionnaire asked,
among other things, whether the resident's clinical work had
been supervised by an impaired psychiatrist. In order to minimize possible confusion about the term *impairment,* Igartua
provided a definition proposed by the American Medical Association's Council on Mental Health: "inability to practice medicine adequately by reason of physical or mental illness, including alcoholism or drug dependence" [3, p. 684].

Two hundred and twenty-nine residents returned the questionnaire, for a response rate of 38.2 percent. Seventeen residents (7.4%) reported having worked with impaired supervisors,
and six of those residents said they developed anxiety or depression as a result. The great majority of residents who worked
with impaired supervisors tried to cope with the situation by

doing without supervision, by sharing their feelings, and by seeking supervision from other staff members or senior residents. In addition, almost all of them (15 of 17) felt that other staff were too passive in dealing with the situation. Fourteen of the affected residents were ambivalent about reporting their supervisors, but 12 of them did so.

Igartua understood the methodological limitations of her study, but she also saw its potential implications: "The low response rate (38%) makes it difficult to draw conclusions. However, if we presuppose that none of the nonresponders had worked with impaired supervisors, the risk of working with an impaired supervisor during residency training would be 4%" [90, p. 192]. Had Kozlowska and her colleagues made the same assumption, the risk of working with an impaired supervisor during training would be about 19 percent. If the risk for residents in general is somewhere between those two figures, and if you are in a residency program of average size, the chances are that at least one of your colleagues has an impaired supervisor.

Sexual Harassment by a Supervisor

The concept of sexual harassment includes behaviors that are gender-related, unwanted, and occur in a context where one person has power over another [10, p. S6]. Such behaviors can be verbal (e.g., making a sexist joke, commenting on someone's dress or physique, making a sexual proposition) or nonverbal (e.g., using offensive body language, touching). Although there have been many surveys of sexual harassment experienced by medical students and house officers in general, none has focused on psychiatry residents and their psychotherapy supervisors. In some studies, such as those by Deborah Cook and her colleagues [29] and Steven Daugherty and his colleagues [34], psychiatry residents were included among the house officers surveyed, but the results were not analyzed by specialty. And although Kozlowska and her colleagues assessed sexual harassment in their survey of adverse experiences for psychiatry trainees [101], it is not clear to what extent the harassment was perpetrated by peers, senior psychiatrists, nurses, or other staff.

To my knowledge, only one survey specifically investigated the sexual harassment of psychiatry residents by their teachers. In that study, Melanie Carr and her colleagues sent a self-report questionnaire to all 535 residents enrolled in Canadian programs [25]. Three hundred fourteen questionnaires were returned, for a response rate of 58.7 percent. The respondents included 169 males and 145 females. Two hundred and ninety-six of them (94.3%) described themselves as heterosexual, 13 (4.1%) as homosexual, and five (1.6%) as bisexual. Eighty-two residents were in the PGY-1 year, 76 in the PGY-2 year, 68 in the PGY-3 year, and 88 in the PGY-4 year.

Although the major focus of the survey was sexual involvement of residents with their teachers (see below), the investigators also asked about sexual harassment. A teacher ("psychiatric educator") was defined as a clinical supervisor, a course instructor, an advisor, or a residency program administrator; the term *sexual harassment* was not defined. Twenty-one of the 314 respondents (6.7%) reported that they had been propositioned by a teacher. Of this group, 19 were females (13.1% of female respondents) and two were males (1.2% of male respondents). In addition, 14 female respondents (9.7%) said that they had been sexually harassed by a teacher, whereas no male respondents did.

When a teacher violates the boundaries of the student-teacher relationship, the student is often upset and uncertain what to do next. The distressing and complicated nature of this situation is illustrated in the study conducted by Deborah Cook and her colleagues of all residents in programs sponsored by McMaster University during the 1993–1994 academic year [29]. The investigators surveyed 225 residents in seven programs (anesthesia, family medicine, internal medicine, obstetrics and gynecology, pediatrics, psychiatry, and surgery) about a variety of topics, including sexual harassment. One hundred and eighty-six residents (82.7%) returned the questionnaire, with response rates ranging from 69.0 percent for family medicine to 100 percent for anesthesia and internal medicine. The rates were almost equal for male and female residents: for males, 93 of 111 (83.8%); for females, 93 of 114 (81.6%).

One hundred and eighty-four residents completed at least some of the questions regarding 14 events the investigators thought could be experienced as sexual harassment. One hundred and seventy-one of these residents (92.9%) reported experiencing one or more such events, the most common of which were sexist jokes, compliments on the resident's physique, flirtation, and body language deemed offensive. More male residents (11.0%) than female residents (6.5%) reported having been made an explicit sexual proposition, but the difference was not statistically significant. There was no relationship between the type of residency program and the frequency of any of the 14 events. The investigators did not ask the respondents to identify the type of person (e.g., supervising physician, resident, nurse, other staff member, patient, patient's relative) responsible for the event.

One hundred and fifty-four residents described their emotional responses to these events. The most common reactions were embarrassment (24.0%), anger (23.4%), frustration (20.8%), anxiety (16.2%), feeling violated (11.0%), and helplessness (7.1%). Significantly more females than males reported feelings of anger, frustration, violation, and helplessness, whereas significantly more males than females stated that the events had made no emotional impact on them.

Of the 171 residents who reported events defined as sexual harassment, 165 answered the question that dealt with whether they had told anyone about the event. Seventy-nine of these 165 (47.9%) stated they had, and 78 of them indicated whom they had told. The most common confidants were other residents (70.5% of cases), friends (65.4%), partners or family members (53.8%), and supervising physicians (23.1%).

When respondents were asked why they had not made a formal complaint about the most distressing event they had experienced, 123 provided reasons. Most often, it was because they did not consider the behavior in question to be a problem (45.5% of cases), because they thought it was too small a problem to worry about (30.9%), because they believed that making a formal complaint would not accomplish anything (25.2%), because they thought that complaining was more trouble than it was worth (18.7%), or because they feared that complaining would adversely affect their evaluations (13.8%). Seventeen of the 123 (13.8%) said they did not make a formal complaint of sexual harassment because they had dealt with the matter themselves.

The survey conducted by Cook and her colleagues illustrates not only how distressing and complicated it can be for residents to deal with sexual harassment, but also how residents (among others) can disagree about what sexual harassment is. Although Cook and her colleagues listed 14 events as examples of sexual harassment, it seems that many of the residents who experienced some of those events did not regard them as such. Thus, certain residents might have thought that a sexist joke was gauche or boorish behavior but not sexual harassment.

If you believe a teacher's conduct toward you is sexual harassment, your decision to confront the teacher or tell your residency director will probably depend on several factors. You may be less likely to protest, for example, if the behavior is a single offensive joke than if it is a repeated sexual proposition; you may be less likely to protest if you are a forgiving or passive person than if you are a censorious or assertive one; and you may be less likely to protest if you have a distant relationship with your residency director than if you have a close one.

I urge you to confide in your residency director if you have been sexually harassed by a teacher or if you are uncertain whether a teacher's behavior constitutes sexual harassment. It is much more likely that you will be hurt by the unwanted comments, propositions, or actions of someone whose behavior should merit your respect (a category of persons that includes other residents as well as teachers) than it is that you will be hurt by reporting misconduct to someone who is responsible for your welfare as a resident.

Sexual Involvement with a Supervisor

Although sexual harassment of residents by psychotherapy supervisors can be unequivocally condemned because it is unwanted and imposed, what if a resident and supervisor establish a sexual relationship by mutual consent? Do you believe that, given the power differential between students and teachers, the resident cannot be an equal partner in the relationship, or do you believe that two adults may do as they wish, even if one happens to be the pupil of the other? Questions such as these prompted three groups of investigators to survey psychiatry residents about sexual involvement with their teachers.

The first of these studies, by Nanette Gartrell and her colleagues [57], was based on a self-report questionnaire sent to all 1,113 PGY-4 residents listed in the 1986 American Medical Association Physician Masterfile. Of the 1,087 questionnaires that were delivered, 548 (50.4%) were returned, though not all respondents answered every question. Three hundred and twenty-one respondents (58.6%) were male, 225 (41.1%) were female, and two (0.4%) did not specify their sex. Relatively more female residents (57.7%) than male residents (44.4%) returned the questionnaire.

The major focus of the survey was on sexual involvement of residents with their teachers, but it also asked about sexual involvement of residents with their patients. As I noted in chapter 3, 0.9 percent of the respondents acknowledged having been sexually involved with patients. In what follows, I will summarize the findings of the survey in relation to residents' sexual involvement with teachers. The investigators defined sexual involvement ("sexual contact") as behavior "intended to arouse or satisfy sexual desire" [p. 691]. They defined a teacher ("psychiatric educator") as a clinical supervisor, a course instructor, an advisor, or a residency program administrator. (These two definitions were subsequently used by Melanie Carr and her colleagues in their survey of Canadian psychiatry residents—a survey whose findings on sexual harassment were summarized above and whose findings on sexual relationships with teachers are summarized below.)

Gartrell and her colleagues found that almost three-quarters (74.2%) of the respondents in their survey believed that sexual involvement with a current teacher was inappropriate, but even more (80.0%) believed that such involvement could be appropriate if the resident and teacher did not have an ongoing work relationship. Male and female respondents were of the same opinion in regard to these issues.

As to the question of whether they had been sexually involved with their teachers, 26 (4.9%) of 527 respondents acknowledged that they had. (See table 5.) Fourteen of these residents were female (6.3% of female respondents) and 12 were male (3.9% of male respondents). In 14 cases, the sexual contact occurred between female residents and male teachers; in nine cases, between male residents and female teachers; in two cases, between male residents and male teachers; and in one case the respondent did not specify the sex of either party. The contact was initiated more often by the teacher when the resident was female (9 of 14 cases) than when the resident was male (2 of 11 cases).

Sexual involvement of residents with teachers often occurred early in the resident's training. Of the twenty-two respondents who specified when the involvement began, seven were in the PGY-1 year, five were in the PGY-2 year, eight were in the PGY-3 year, and two were in the PGY-4 year. Only 12 respondents identified the role of the teacher at the time: in seven cases it was as a clinical supervisor; in two cases, as a course instructor; in two cases, as an administrator; and in one case, as an advisor. In 11 cases the involvement began during a work relationship; in 14 cases it did not; and in one case the respondent did not answer the question.

Respondents were asked what they thought about the involvement at the time it occurred and were permitted to give multiple answers to this question. More respondents believed the relationship was "appropriate" (16), "caring" (11), or "helpful" (3) than believed it was "inappropriate" (2), "exploitative" (2), or "harmful" (1). When asked what they thought about the involvement at the time they filled out the questionnaire, fewer residents believed it had been "appropriate" (9), "caring" (8), or "helpful" (3), and more believed it had been "inappropriate" (7), "exploitative" (7), or "harmful" (7). At the time they filled out the questionnaire, 13 respondents were no longer sexually involved with their teachers, seven were, and six did not answer the ques-

Table 5. Surveys of Sexual Involvement of Residents with Teachers

Authors; Publication Date	Number and Source of Potential Respondents	Response Rate (%)	Rate of Residents' Sexual Involvement (%)
Gartrell et al. 1988 [57]	All 1,113 PGY-4 residents in 1986 AMA Physician Masterfile	50.4	4.9
Carr et al. 1991 [25]	All 535 Canadian psychiatry residents	58.7	2.5
Kozlowska et al. 1997 [101]	All 137 house officers in New South Wales with at least one year of training; all 95 consultant psychiatrists in New South Wales certified within last five years	76.7	2.8

Abbreviations: AMA = American Medical Association

tion. Four of the respondents were currently married to the teachers with whom they had been involved.

In the second survey of sexual involvement of psychiatry residents with their teachers, Melanie Carr and her colleagues sent a self-report questionnaire to all 535 residents enrolled in Canadian programs [25]. Three hundred and fourteen questionnaires were returned, for a response rate of 58.7 percent. The respondents included 169 males and 145 females. Two hundred and ninety-six of them (94.3%) described themselves as heterosexual, 13 (4.1%) as homosexual, and five (1.6%) as bisexual. Eighty-two residents were in the PGY-1 year, 76 in the PGY-2 year, 68 in the PGY-3 year, and 88 in the PGY-4 year.

Seventy respondents (22.3%) thought that sexual involvement of residents with teachers was unethical under any circumstances; 11 (3.5%) thought it was permissible in special circumstances (a concept not defined in the paper); eight (2.5%) thought it was permissible outside of supervisory sessions; 80 (25.5%) thought it was permissible if the teacher was not a direct supervisor; and 115 (36.6%) thought it was permissible if the supervisory relationship had been terminated. The investigators did not comment on the responses of the remaining 30 residents (9.6%).

Eight respondents (2.5%) acknowledged a total of nine sexual relationships with their teachers. (See table 5.) Six of those residents were female (4.1% of female respondents) and two were male (1.2% of male respondents). One of the female residents reported having had sexual relationships with two teachers. All of the relationships were heterosexual.

At the time of the involvement, one resident was in the PGY-1 year; two in the PGY-2 year; two in the PGY-3 year; and three in the PGY-4 year. In five cases, the teacher was the resident's supervisor, and in two of these cases the teacher was also the resident's psychotherapy supervisor. In the remaining three cases the teacher's role was not specified.

In five of the nine relationships, the sexual involvement was mutually initiated; in four of the relationships, it was initiated by the teacher. Information about the duration of the involvement was reported for seven relationships: in two, it was limited to a single contact; in four, it lasted three months; and in one, it lasted three years and resulted in marriage.

At the time the respondents filled out the questionnaire, four were no longer in contact with the teachers; one had a work relationship but no sexual involvement; two had sexual involvement but no work relationship; and two had both sexual involvement and a work relationship. Looking back on the sexual involvement with their teachers, six of the respondents had positive feelings, one had mixed feelings (i.e., that the relationship had been caring but harmful and inappropriate), and one had neutral feelings. Five of the respondents had not told anyone of their involvement; three had told friends. None of the eight respondents who had been sexually involved with their teachers expressed any regrets.

The third survey of sexual involvement of psychiatry residents with their teachers was conducted in 1994 by Kasia Kozlowska and her colleagues in Australia [100; 101]. Some of the results of that survey, which assessed many aspects of a resident's experience with patients, teachers, and peers, are summarized above in the section on impaired supervisors.

Kozlowska and her colleagues sent a self-report questionnaire to all 137 house officers in New South Wales who had completed at least one year of training, and to all 95 consultants (the equivalent of board-certified psychiatrists) in New South Wales who had achieved specialist status within the previous five years. Of the 232 questionnaires sent out, 178 (76.7%) were completed and returned: 110 of them from trainees (response rate: 80.3%) and 68 from consultants (response rate: 71.6%).

Of the 178 respondents, five (2.8%) acknowledged a sexual relationship with a senior colleague. (See table 5.) Other than noting that all of the respondents involved were female, that one of the relationships ended in marriage, and that another relationship contributed to the respondent's decision to leave psychiatry, the investigators provided no other information, perhaps because their survey was so wide-ranging that they had to sacrifice depth of inquiry for breadth.

These three surveys suggest that it is relatively uncommon for psychiatry residents to become sexually involved with their supervisors. The question remains, however, whether such relationships ought to be seen as acceptable or unacceptable. Kozlowska and her colleagues did not attempt to answer the question, but the other groups of investigators did. For both of them, the sexual involvement of residents and supervisors was a matter not only of student-teacher relationships but also of professional responsibility. Gartrell and her colleagues took an unambiguous position on the question: "Sexual contact between a psychiatric educator and resident is unethical as long as the educator has authority over the resident. We recognize that such authority may be of long duration, continuing as long as the educator is in a position to advance or obstruct the student's professional career" [57, p. 694]. Carr and her colleagues were less direct in their disapproval, but their conclusion was clear: "Departmental policies concerning sexual contact are necessary to ensure the protection of residents during the vulnerable training period. Above all, professional integrity and ethical accountability are not only learned through the intellectual examination of issues but incorporated by example. The supervisory relationship in resident education deserves careful scrutiny in this regard" [25, p. 219].

The American Psychiatric Association's publication *The Principles of Medical Ethics with Annotations Especially Applicable to Psychiatry* does not prohibit sexual relationships between residents and supervisors, but it does warn against them:

> Sexual involvement between a faculty member or supervisor and a trainee or student, in those situations in which an abuse of power can occur, often takes advantage of inequalities in the working relationship and may be unethical because—
> a. Any treatment of a patient being supervised may be deleteriously affected.
> b. It may damage the trust relationship between teacher and student.
> c. Teachers are important professional role models for their trainees and affect their trainees' future professional behavior. [6, p. 9]

Given the vulnerability of some residents to exploitation and the tendency of some psychiatrists to take advantage of those (whether patients or students) for whom they have responsibility, such warnings are appropriate. Still, residents are adults, and adults are presumed to be competent to choose their own relationships. This position was vigorously advanced by Christopher Ryan, who grounded his argument in the principle of autonomy, but even Ryan found two reasons to condemn the sexual involvement of psychiatry residents with current supervisors:

The first concerns the psychiatrist's role as a supervisor. The psychiatrist-supervisor has a primary role in shaping the trainee's development and reporting to the training body regarding the trainee's progress. A supervisor's ability to complete these tasks will be impaired if they are, or have been, their trainee's lover. . . . A supervisor involved in a sexual relationship with a trainee will not be able to give dispassionate and effective feedback either to the training body or to the trainee. . . .

There is also the possibility that a sexual relationship may result in harm to patients under the care of the trainee that the psychiatrist is supervising. The supervisor may be less able to identify mistakes made by the trainee. In addition, the trainee may be more likely to withhold information concerning adverse events in their therapeutic contacts so as to appear to their supervisor in a better light. [150, pp. 387–88]

Psychotherapy supervision is a delicate process for both student and teacher: the former must trust and take risks; the latter, encourage and criticize. All of this is hard enough without sexual involvement. If you and your psychotherapy supervisor find one another so attractive that you cannot postpone a romantic relationship until you are no longer working together, I suggest that both of you discuss the matter with your residency director and department director. This discussion will either facilitate the relationship (e.g., by assigning you another supervisor, by changing your rotation schedule) or make it clear that such relationships are frowned upon or proscribed. If a secret romantic relationship goes badly, with negative consequences for you, your supervisor, or your patients, the residency director and department director may be less sympathetic than if they had known about the relationship beforehand.

Epilogue

Becoming a psychotherapist takes practice, supervision, and patience. You must learn to balance engagement and detachment. Theory and technique are important, but they are less important than common sense and character.

Although much depends on you, patients who do not apply themselves will not improve. Psychotherapy is more like rehabilitation medicine than it is like surgery.

Becoming a psychotherapist, like becoming a physician, means learning to deal with failure. And even when a course of psychotherapy has a happy ending, there may be times when your confidence falters and you cannot sleep because you fear you have made a mistake. I have been a psychotherapist for more than thirty years, but I still ask my colleagues for advice.

Psychotherapy is the most personal of treatments, for both you and your patients. As such, it is a risky business. Listen before you speak. Think before you act. It is precisely because psychotherapy is so personal, so risky, that it can provide such great satisfaction. I wish you well.

References

1. Adler, Alfred. *Problems of Neurosis.* Edited by Philippe Mairet. With a prefatory essay by F. G. Crookshank. New York: Cosmopolitan Book Corporation, 1930.

2. Alden, Lynn. "Short-Term Structured Treatment for Avoidant Personality Disorder." *Journal of Consulting and Clinical Psychology* 57 (1989): 756–64.

3. American Medical Association, Council on Mental Health. "The Sick Physician: Impairment by Psychiatric Disorders, Including Alcoholism and Drug Dependence." *Journal of the American Medical Association* 223 (1973): 684–87.

4. American Psychiatric Association. *Census of Psychiatry Residents: 2001–2002.* Arlington, VA: American Psychiatric Association, 2003.

5. American Psychiatric Association. *Diagnostic and Statistical Manual of Mental Disorders.* 4th ed. Washington, DC: American Psychiatric Association, 1994.

6. American Psychiatric Association. *The Principles of Medical Ethics: With Annotations Especially Applicable to Psychiatry.* Washington, DC: American Psychiatric Association, 2001.

7. Appelbaum, Paul S., and Jorgenson, Linda. "Psychotherapist-Patient Sexual Contact after Termination of Treatment: An Analysis and a Proposal." *American Journal of Psychiatry* 148 (1991): 1466–73.

8. Appelbaum, Paul S.; Jorgenson, Linda M.; and Sutherland, Pamela K. "Sexual Relationships between Physicians and Patients." *Archives of Internal Medicine* 154 (1994): 2561–65.

9. Bachrach, Henry M. "Empathy: We Know What We Mean, But What Do We Measure?" *Archives of General Psychiatry* 33 (1976): 35–38.

10. Baldwin, DeWitt C., Jr., and Daugherty, Steven R. "Distinguishing Sexual Harassment from Discrimination: A Factor-Analytic Study of Residents' Reports." *Academic Medicine*, October Supplement (2001).

11. Barber, Jacques P.; Connolly, Mary Beth; Crits-Christoph,

Paul; Gladis, Lynn; and Siqueland, Lynne. "Alliance Predicts Patients' Outcome Beyond In-Treatment Change in Symptoms." *Journal of Consulting and Clinical Psychology* 68 (2000): 1027–32.

12. Bateman, Anthony W., and Fonagy, Peter. "Effectiveness of Psychotherapeutic Treatment of Personality Disorder." *British Journal of Psychiatry* 177 (2000): 138–43.

13. Bayer, Timothy; Coverdale, John; and Chiang, Elizabeth. "A National Survey of Physicians' Behaviors regarding Sexual Contact with Patients." *Southern Medical Journal* 89 (1996): 977–82.

14. Berland, David I., and Guskin, Karen. "Patient Allegations of Sexual Abuse against Psychiatric Hospital Staff." *General Hospital Psychiatry* 16 (1994): 335–39.

15. Bernstein, David P.; Kasapis, Chrysoula; Bergman, Andrea; Weld, Ellen; Mitropoulou, Vivian; Horvath, Thomas; Klar, Howard M.; Silverman, Jeremy; and Siever, Larry J. "Assessing Axis II Disorders by Informant Interview." *Journal of Personality Disorders* 11 (1997): 158–67.

16. Betcher, R. William, and Zinberg, Norman E. "Supervision and Privacy in Psychotherapy Training." *American Journal of Psychiatry* 145 (1988): 796–803.

17. Beutler, Larry E.; Machado, Paulo P. P.; and Neufeldt, Susan Allstetter. "Therapist Variables." In *Handbook of Psychotherapy and Behavior Change,* 4th ed., edited by Allen E. Bergin and Sol L. Garfield, 229–69. New York: John Wiley and Sons, 1994.

18. Blatt, Sidney J. "Commentary: The Therapeutic Process and Professional Boundary Guidelines." *Journal of the American Academy of Psychiatry and the Law* 29 (2001): 290–93.

19. Bordin, Edward S. "The Generalizability of the Psychoanalytic Concept of the Working Alliance." *Psychotherapy: Theory, Research and Practice* 16 (1979): 252–60.

20. Borus, Jonathan F. "Economics and Psychiatric Education: The Irresistible Force Meets the Moveable Object." *Harvard Review of Psychiatry* 2 (1994): 15–21.

21. Bouhoutsos, Jacqueline; Holroyd, Jean; Lerman, Hannah; Forer, Bertram R.; and Greenberg, Mimi. "Sexual Intimacy between Psychotherapists and Patients." *Professional Psychology: Research and Practice* 14 (1983): 185–96.

22. Breuer, Josef. "Fräulein Anna O." In *The Standard Edition of the Complete Psychological Works of Sigmund Freud.* Translated and

edited by James Strachey, 2:21–47. 1955. 24 vols. London: Hogarth Press and the Institute of Psycho-Analysis, 1953–74.

23. Bruch, Hilde. *Learning Psychotherapy: Rationale and Ground Rules*. Cambridge, MA: Harvard University Press, 1974.

24. Carney, Francis L. "Outpatient Treatment of the Aggressive Offender." *American Journal of Psychotherapy* 31 (1977): 265–74.

25. Carr, Melanie L.; Robinson, G. Erlick; Stewart, Donna E.; and Kussin, Dennis. "A Survey of Canadian Psychiatric Residents regarding Resident-Educator Sexual Contact." *American Journal of Psychiatry* 148 (1991): 216–20.

26. Chessick, Richard D. "Psychoanalytic Peregrinations I: Transference and Transference Neurosis Revisited." *Journal of the American Academy of Psychoanalysis* 30 (2002): 83–97.

27. Childress, Robert, and Gillis, John S. "A Study of Pretherapy Role Induction as an Influence Process." *Journal of Clinical Psychology* 33 (1977): 540–44.

28. Cleckley, Hervey. *The Mask of Sanity: An Attempt to Clarify Some Issues about the So-Called Psychopathic Personality*. 4th ed. St. Louis: C. V. Mosby, 1964.

29. Cook, Deborah J.; Liutkus, Joanne F.; Risdon, Catherine L.; Griffith, Lauren E.; Guyatt, Gordon H.; and Walter, Stephen D. "Residents' Experiences of Abuse, Discrimination and Sexual Harassment during Residency Training." *Canadian Medical Association Journal* 154 (1996): 1657–65.

30. Costa, Paul T., Jr., and McCrae, Robert R. *Revised NEO Personality Inventory (NEO PI-R) and NEO Five-Factor Inventory (NEO-FFI): Professional Manual*. Odessa, FL: Psychological Assessment Resources, 1992.

31. Coverdale, John; Bayer, Timothy; Chiang, Elizabeth; Thornby, John; and Bangs, Mark. "National Survey on Physicians' Attitudes toward Social and Sexual Contact with Patients." *Southern Medical Journal* 87 (1994): 1067–71.

32. Coverdale, John H.; Thomson, Alex N.; and White, Gillian E. "Social and Sexual Contact between General Practitioners and Patients in New Zealand: Attitudes and Prevalence." *British Journal of General Practice* 45 (1995): 245–47.

33. Daly, Karen A. "Attitudes of U.S. Psychiatry Residencies about Personal Psychotherapy for Psychiatry Residents." *Academic Psychiatry* 22 (1998): 223–28.

34. Daugherty, Steven R.; Baldwin, DeWitt C., Jr.; and Rowley, Beverley D. "Learning, Satisfaction, and Mistreatment during Medical Internship: A National Survey of Working Conditions." *Journal of the American Medical Association* 279 (1998): 1194–99.

35. de Figueiredo, John M., and Frank, Jerome D. "Subjective Incompetence, the Clinical Hallmark of Demoralization." *Comprehensive Psychiatry* 23 (1982): 353–63.

36. Dunn, Jocelyn J.; Lee, Thomas H.; Percelay, Jack M.; Fitz, J. Gregory; and Goldman, Lee. "Patient and House Officer Attitudes on Physician Attire and Etiquette." *Journal of the American Medical Association* 257 (1987): 65–68.

37. Edelstein, Ludwig. "The Hippocratic Oath: Text, Translation and Interpretation." *Bulletin of the History of Medicine,* Supplement 1 (1943).

38. Eysenck, H. J. "Personality and Drug Effects." In *Experiments with Drugs: Studies in the Relation between Personality, Learning Theory and Drug Action,* edited by H. J. Eysenck, 1–24. Oxford: Pergamon Press, 1963.

39. Fenton, Lisa R.; Cecero, John J.; Nich, Charla; Frankforter, Tami L.; and Carroll, Kathleen M. "Perspective Is Everything: The Predictive Validity of Six Working Alliance Instruments." *Journal of Psychotherapy Practice and Research* 10 (2001): 262–68.

40. Fiedler, Fred E. "A Comparison of Therapeutic Relationships in Psychoanalytic, Nondirective and Adlerian Therapy." *Journal of Consulting Psychology* 14 (1950): 436–45.

41. Fiedler, Fred E. "The Concept of an Ideal Therapeutic Relationship." *Journal of Consulting Psychology* 14 (1950): 239–45.

42. Frances, Allen. "Categorical and Dimensional Systems of Personality Diagnosis: A Comparison." *Comprehensive Psychiatry* 23 (1982): 516–27.

43. Frank, Jerome D. "Psychotherapists Need Theories." *International Journal of Psychiatry* 9 (1970–1971): 146–49.

44. Frank, Jerome D., and Frank, Julia B. *Persuasion and Healing: A Comparative Study of Psychotherapy.* 3d ed. Baltimore: Johns Hopkins University Press, 1991.

45. Freud, Sigmund. "The Future Prospects of Psycho-Analytic Therapy." In *The Standard Edition of the Complete Psychological Works of Sigmund Freud.* Translated and edited by James Strachey, 11:139–51. 1964. 24 vols. London: Hogarth Press and the Institute of Psycho-Analysis, 1953–74.

46. Freud, Sigmund. "The Interpretation of Dreams." In *Standard Edition*, 4. 1953. *See* 45.

47. Freud, Sigmund. "On Beginning the Treatment (Further Recommendations on the Technique of Psycho-Analysis I)." In *Standard Edition*, 12:121–44. 1958. *See* 45.

48. Freud, Sigmund. "On the History of the Psycho-Analytic Movement." In *Standard Edition*, 14:7–66. 1957. *See* 45.

49. Freud, Sigmund. "The Psychotherapy of Hysteria." In *Standard Edition*, 2:253–305. 1955. *See* 45.

50. Freud, Sigmund. "Recommendations to Physicians Practising Psycho-Analysis." In *Standard Edition*, 12:109–20. 1958. *See* 45.

51. Gabbard, Glen O. "Commentary: Boundaries, Culture, and Psychotherapy." *Journal of the American Academy of Psychiatry and the Law* 29 (2001): 284–86.

52. Gabbard, Glen O. "A Contemporary Psychoanalytic Model of Countertransference." *Journal of Clinical Psychology/In Session* 57 (2001): 983–91.

53. Gabbard, Glen O. "Post-Termination Sexual Boundary Violations." *Psychiatric Clinics of North America* 25 (2002): 593–603.

54. Gabbard, Glen O. "Psychotherapy of Personality Disorders." *Journal of Psychotherapy Practice and Research* 9 (2000): 1–6.

55. Garfield, Sol L., and Bergin, Allen E. "Personal Therapy, Outcome and Some Therapist Variables." *Psychotherapy: Theory, Research and Practice* 8 (1971): 251–53.

56. Gartrell, Nanette; Herman, Judith; Olarte, Silvia; Feldstein, Michael; and Localio, Russell. "Psychiatrist-Patient Sexual Contact: Results of a National Survey, I: Prevalence." *American Journal of Psychiatry* 143 (1986): 1126–31.

57. Gartrell, Nanette; Herman, Judith; Olarte, Silvia; Localio, Russell; and Feldstein, Michael. "Psychiatric Residents' Sexual Contact with Educators and Patients: Results of a National Survey." *American Journal of Psychiatry* 145 (1988): 690–94.

58. Gartrell, Nanette K.; Milliken, Nancy; Goodson, William H., III; Thiemann, Sue; and Lo, Bernard. "Physician-Patient Sexual Contact: Prevalence and Problems." *Western Journal of Medicine* 157 (1992): 139–43.

59. Gass, Carlton S. "Therapeutic Influence as a Function of Therapist Attire and the Seating Arrangement in an Initial Interview." *Journal of Clinical Psychology* 40 (1984): 52–57.

60. Gaston, Louise. "The Concept of the Alliance and Its Role in

Psychotherapy: Theoretical and Empirical Considerations." *Psychotherapy* 27 (1990): 143–53.

61. Gledhill, Julia A.; Warner, James P.; and King, Michael. "Psychiatrists and Their Patients: Views on Forms of Dress and Address." *British Journal of Psychiatry* 171 (1997): 228–32.

62. Goethe, Johann Wolfgang von. *Wilhelm Meister's Apprenticeship*. Translated and edited by Eric A. Blackall in cooperation with Victor Lange. Princeton, NJ: Princeton University Press, 1994.

63. Gorton, Gregg E., and Samuel, Steven E. "A National Survey of Training Directors about Education for Prevention of Psychiatrist-Patient Sexual Exploitation." *Academic Psychiatry* 20 (1996): 92–98.

64. Gorton, Gregg E.; Samuel, Steven E.; and Zebrowski, Sandra M. "A Pilot Course for Residents on Sexual Feelings and Boundary Maintenance in Treatment." *Academic Psychiatry* 20 (1996): 43–55.

65. Greben, Stanley E. "On Being Therapeutic." *Canadian Psychiatric Association Journal* 22 (1977): 371–80.

66. Greben, Stanley E. "Interpersonal Aspects of the Supervision of Individual Psychotherapy." *American Journal of Psychotherapy* 45 (1991): 306–16.

67. Greenspan, Marie, and Kulish, Nancy Mann. "Factors in Premature Termination in Long-Term Psychotherapy." *Psychotherapy* 22 (1985): 75–82.

68. Group for the Advancement of Psychiatry, Committee on Medical Education. *Trends and Issues in Psychiatry Residency Programs*. Report no. 31. Topeka, KS: Group for the Advancement of Psychiatry, 1955.

69. Gunderson, John G. *Borderline Personality Disorder: A Clinical Guide*. Washington, DC: American Psychiatric Publishing, 2001.

70. Gutheil, Thomas G. "Borderline Personality Disorder, Boundary Violations, and Patient-Therapist Sex: Medicolegal Pitfalls." *American Journal of Psychiatry* 146 (1989): 597–602.

71. Gutheil, Thomas G., and Gabbard, Glen O. "The Concept of Boundaries in Clinical Practice: Theoretical and Risk-Management Dimensions." *American Journal of Psychiatry* 150 (1993): 188–96.

72. Gutheil, Thomas G., and Gabbard, Glen O. "Misuses and Misunderstandings of Boundary Theory in Clinical and Regulatory Settings." *American Journal of Psychiatry* 155 (1998): 409–14.

73. Gutheil, Thomas G., and Simon, Robert I. "Non-Sexual

Boundary Crossings and Boundary Violations: The Ethical Dimension." *Psychiatric Clinics of North America* 25 (2002): 585–92.

74. Hantoot, Mark S. "Lying in Psychotherapy Supervision: Why Residents Say One Thing and Do Another." *Academic Psychiatry* 24 (2000): 179–87.

75. Heider, Fritz, and Simmel, Marianne. "An Experimental Study of Apparent Behavior." *American Journal of Psychology* 57 (1944): 243–59.

76. Heimann, Paula. "On Counter-Transference." *International Journal of Psycho-Analysis* 31 (1950): 81–84.

77. Heine, Ralph W., ed. *The Student Physician as Psychotherapist.* Chicago: University of Chicago Press, 1962.

78. Henry, William P., and Strupp, Hans H. "The Therapeutic Alliance as Interpersonal Process." In *The Working Alliance: Theory, Research, and Practice,* edited by Adam O. Horvath and Leslie S. Greenberg, 51–84. New York: John Wiley and Sons, 1994.

79. Henry, William P.; Strupp, Hans H.; Schacht, Thomas E.; and Gaston, Louise. "Psychodynamic Approaches." In *Handbook of Psychotherapy and Behavior Change,* 4th ed., edited by Allen E. Bergin and Sol L. Garfield, 467–508. New York: John Wiley and Sons, 1994.

80. Herman, Judith Lewis; Gartrell, Nanette; Olarte, Silvia; Feldstein, Michael; and Localio, Russell. "Psychiatrist-Patient Sexual Contact: Results of a National Survey, II: Psychiatrists' Attitudes." *American Journal of Psychiatry* 144 (1987): 164–69.

81. Hill, A. B. "Extraversion and Variety-Seeking in a Monotonous Task." *British Journal of Psychology* 66 (1975): 9–13.

82. Hoehn-Saric, Rudolf; Frank, Jerome D.; Imber, Stanley D.; Nash, Earl H.; Stone, Anthony R.; and Battle, Carolyn C. "Systematic Preparation of Patients for Psychotherapy—I. Effects on Therapy Behavior and Outcome." *Journal of Psychiatric Research* 2 (1964): 267–81.

83. Hoge, Michael A.; Jacobs, Selby C.; and Belitsky, Richard. "Psychiatric Residency Training, Managed Care, and Contemporary Clinical Practice." *Psychiatric Services* 51 (2000): 1001–5.

84. Hollender, Marc H. "The Case of Anna O: A Reformulation." *American Journal of Psychiatry* 137 (1980): 797–800.

85. Holroyd, Jean Corey, and Brodsky, Annette M. "Psychologists' Attitudes and Practices Regarding Erotic and Nonerotic Physical Contact with Patients." *American Psychologist* 32 (1977): 843–49.

86. Horowitz, Mardi J. "Psychotherapy for Histrionic Personal-

ity Disorder." *Journal of Psychotherapy Practice and Research* 6 (1997): 93–107.

87. Horvath, Adam O. "Research on the Alliance." In *The Working Alliance: Theory, Research, and Practice,* edited by Adam O. Horvath and Leslie S. Greenberg, 259–86. New York: John Wiley and Sons, 1994.

88. Horvath, Adam O. "The Therapeutic Relationship: From Transference to Alliance." *Journal of Clinical Psychology/In Session* 56 (2000): 163–73.

89. Horvath, Adam O., and Symonds, B. Dianne. "Relation between Working Alliance and Outcome in Psychotherapy: A Meta-Analysis." *Journal of Counseling Psychology* 38 (1991): 139–49.

90. Igartua, Karine J. "The Impact of Impaired Supervisors on Residents." *Academic Psychiatry* 24 (2000): 188–94.

91. Jaspers, Karl. *General Psychopathology.* Translated by J. Hoenig and Marian W. Hamilton. With a new foreword by Paul R. McHugh. 2 vols. Baltimore: Johns Hopkins University Press, 1997.

92. Kardener, Sheldon H.; Fuller, Marielle; and Mensh, Ivan N. "A Survey of Physicians' Attitudes and Practices regarding Erotic and Nonerotic Contact with Patients." *American Journal of Psychiatry* 130 (1973): 1077–81.

93. Katz, Martin M.; Lorr, Maurice; and Rubinstein, Eli A. "Remainer Patient Attributes and Their Relation to Subsequent Improvement in Psychotherapy." *Journal of Consulting Psychology* 22 (1958): 411–13.

94. Kernberg, Otto F. *Borderline Conditions and Pathological Narcissism.* New York: Jason Aronson, 1975.

95. Kernberg, Otto. "Notes on Countertransference." *Journal of the American Psychoanalytic Association* 13 (1965): 38–56.

96. Kiernan, Kevin W.; Wise, Thomas, N.; and Mann, Lee S. "The Physical Layout of Psychiatric Offices: A Survey." *Psychiatric Journal of the University of Ottawa* 14 (1989): 453–55.

97. Kissane, David W.; Bloch, Sidney; Onghena, Patrick; McKenzie, Dean P.; Snyder, Ray D.; and Dowe, David L. "The Melbourne Family Grief Study, II: Psychosocial Morbidity and Grief in Bereaved Families." *American Journal of Psychiatry* 153 (1996): 659–66.

98. Kohut, Heinz. "The Two Analyses of Mr. Z." *International Journal of Psycho-Analysis* 60 (1979): 3–27.

99. Korb, Margaret P.; Gorrell, Jeffrey; and Van De Riet, Vernon.

Gestalt Therapy: Practice and Theory. 2d ed. New York: Pergamon Press, 1989.

100. Kozlowska, Kasia; Nunn, Kenneth; and Cousens, Penelope. "Training in Psychiatry: An Examination of Trainee Perceptions. Part 1." *Australian and New Zealand Journal of Psychiatry* 31 (1997): 628–40.

101. Kozlowska, Kasia; Nunn, Kenneth; and Cousens, Penelope. "Adverse Experiences in Psychiatric Training. Part 2." *Australian and New Zealand Journal of Psychiatry* 31 (1997): 641–52.

102. Kroll, Jerome. "Boundary Violations: A Culture-Bound Syndrome." *Journal of the American Academy of Psychiatry and the Law* 29 (2001): 274–83.

103. Kroll, Jerome. *The Challenge of the Borderline Patient: Competency in Diagnosis and Treatment.* New York: W. W. Norton, 1988.

104. Krupnick, Janice L.; Sotsky, Stuart M.; Simmens, Sam; Moyer, Janet; Elkin, Irene; Watkins, John; and Pilkonis, Paul A. "The Role of the Therapeutic Alliance in Psychotherapy and Psychotherapy Outcome: Findings in the National Institute of Mental Health Treatment of Depression Collaborative Research Program." *Journal of Consulting and Clinical Psychology* 64 (1996): 532–39.

105. Kuhn, Thomas S. *The Copernican Revolution: Planetary Astronomy in the Development of Western Thought.* Cambridge, MA: Harvard University Press, 1957.

106. Lamont, John A., and Woodward, Christel. "Patient-Physician Sexual Involvement: A Canadian Survey of Obstetrician-Gynecologists." *Canadian Medical Association Journal* 150 (1994): 1433–39.

107. Leggett, Andrew. "A Survey of Australian Psychiatrists' Attitudes and Practices Regarding Physical Contact with Patients." *Australian and New Zealand Journal of Psychiatry* 28 (1994): 488–97.

108. Liberman, Bernard L.; Frank, Jerome D.; Hoehn-Saric, Rudolf; Stone, Anthony R.; Imber, Stanley D.; and Pande, Shashi K. "Patterns of Change in Treated Psychoneurotic Patients: A Five-Year Follow-Up Investigation of the Systematic Preparation of Patients for Psychotherapy." *Journal of Consulting and Clinical Psychology* 38 (1972): 36–41.

109. Livesley, W. John. "Commentary on Reconceptualizing Personality Disorder Categories Using Trait Dimensions." *Journal of Personality* 69 (2001): 277–86.

110. Luborsky, Lester. "Helping Alliances in Psychotherapy." In

Successful Psychotherapy: Proceedings of the Ninth Annual Symposium, November 19–21, 1975, Texas Research Institute of Mental Sciences, edited by James L. Claghorn, 92–116. New York: Brunner/Mazel, 1976.

111. McCrae, Robert R., and Costa, Paul T., Jr. "Personality Trait Structure as a Human Universal." *American Psychologist* 52 (1997): 509–16.

112. McCrae, Robert R., and Costa, Paul T., Jr. "Validation of the Five-Factor Model of Personality across Instruments and Observers." *Journal of Personality and Social Psychology* 52 (1987): 81–90.

113. McCrae, Robert R.; Stone, Stephanie V.; Fagan, Peter J.; and Costa, Paul T., Jr. "Identifying Causes of Disagreement between Self-Reports and Spouse Ratings of Personality." *Journal of Personality* 66 (1998): 285–313.

114. McHugh, Paul R., and Slavney, Phillip R. *The Perspectives of Psychiatry.* 2d ed. Baltimore: Johns Hopkins University Press, 1998.

115. McKendree-Smith, Nancy L.; Floyd, Mark; and Scogin, Forrest R. "Self-Administered Treatments for Depression: A Review." *Journal of Clinical Psychology* 59 (2003): 275–88.

116. McKinstry, Brian, and Wang, Ji-Xiang. "Putting on the Style: What Patients Think of the Way Their Doctor Dresses." *British Journal of General Practice* 41 (1991): 275–78.

117. McNair, Douglas M.; Lorr, Maurice; and Callahan, Daniel M. "Patient and Therapist Influences on Quitting Psychotherapy." *Journal of Consulting Psychology* 27 (1963): 10–17.

118. McNaughton-Filion, Louise; Chen, John S. C.; and Norton, Peter G. "The Physician's Appearance." *Family Medicine* 23 (1991): 208–11.

119. Macaskill, Norman, and Macaskill, Ann. "Psychotherapists-In-Training Evaluate Their Personal Therapy: Results of a UK Study." *British Journal of Psychotherapy* 9 (1992): 133–38.

120. Macran, Susan, and Shapiro, David A. "The Role of Personal Therapy for Therapists: A Review." *British Journal of Medical Psychology* 71 (1998): 13–25.

121. Mains, Jennifer A., and Scogin, Forrest R. "The Effectiveness of Self-Administered Treatments: A Practice-Friendly Review of the Research." *Journal of Clinical Psychology/In Session* 59 (2003): 237–46.

122. Malmquist, Carl P., and Notman, Malkah T. "Psychiatrist-

Patient Boundary Issues following Treatment Termination." *American Journal of Psychiatry* 158 (2001): 1010–18.

123. Marmor, Judd. "Orality in the Hysterical Personality." *Journal of the American Psychoanalytic Association* 1 (1953): 656–71.

124. Marziali, E. "Three Viewpoints on the Therapeutic Alliance: Similarities, Differences, and Associations with Psychotherapy Outcome." *Journal of Nervous and Mental Disease* 172 (1984): 417–23.

125. Millon, Theodore, with Roger D. Davis and contributing associates Carrie M. Millon, Andrew Wenger, Maria H. Van Zuilen, Marketa Fuchs, and Renée B. Millon. *Disorders of Personality: DSM-IV and Beyond.* 2d ed. New York: John Wiley and Sons, 1996.

126. Mitchell, Kevin M.; Bozarth, Jerold D.; and Krauft, Conrad C. "A Reappraisal of the Therapeutic Effectiveness of Accurate Empathy, Nonpossessive Warmth, and Genuineness." In *Effective Psychotherapy: A Handbook of Research,* edited and with commentaries by Alan S. Gurman and Andrew M. Razin, 482–502. Oxford: Pergamon Press, 1977.

127. Moeller, F. Gerard; Dougherty, Donald M.; Lane, Scott D.; Steinberg, Joel L.; and Cherek, Don R. "Antisocial Personality Disorder and Alcohol-Induced Aggression." *Alcoholism: Clinical and Experimental Research* 22 (1998): 1898–1902.

128. Morey, Leslie C.; Gunderson, John; Quigley, Brian D.; and Lyons, Michael. "Dimensions and Categories: The 'Big Five' Factors and the *DSM* Personality Disorders." *Assessment* 7 (2000): 203–16.

129. Nadelson, Carol C.; Belitsky, Catherine; Seeman, Mary V.; and Ablow, Keith. "Gender Issues in Supervision." In *Clinical Perspectives on Psychotherapy Supervision,* edited by Stanley E. Greben and Ronald Ruskin, 41–51. Washington, DC: American Psychiatric Press, 1994.

130. Newman, Michelle G.; Erickson, Thane; Przeworski, Amy; and Dzus, Ellen. "Self-Help and Minimal-Contact Therapies for Anxiety Disorders: Is Human Contact Necessary for Therapeutic Efficacy?" *Journal of Clinical Psychology* 59 (2003): 251–74.

131. Norcross, John C.; Strausser-Kirtland, Dianne; and Missar, C. David. "The Processes and Outcomes of Psychotherapists' Personal Treatment Experiences." *Psychotherapy* 25 (1988): 36–43.

132. Ovens, Howard J., and Permaul-Woods, Joanne A. "Emergency Physicians and Sexual Involvement with Patients: An Ontario Survey." *Canadian Medical Association Journal* 157 (1997): 663–69.

133. Parkes, Colin Murray. "The First Year of Bereavement: A

Longitudinal Study of the Reaction of London Widows to the Death of Their Husbands." *Psychiatry* 33 (1970): 444–67.

134. Peebles, Mary Jo. "Personal Therapy and Ability to Display Empathy, Warmth and Genuineness in Psychotherapy." *Psychotherapy: Theory, Research and Practice* 17 (1980): 258–62.

135. Perls, Fritz. *The Gestalt Approach and Eye Witness to Therapy.* Palo Alto, CA: Science and Behavior Books, 1973.

136. Perry, J. Christopher; Banon, Elisabeth; and Ianni, Floriana. "Effectiveness of Psychotherapy for Personality Disorders." *American Journal of Psychiatry* 156 (1999): 1312–21.

137. Perry, Judith Adams. "Physicians' Erotic and Nonerotic Physical Involvement with Patients." *American Journal of Psychiatry* 133 (1976): 838–40.

138. Pfohl, Bruce; Blum, Nancee; and Zimmerman, Mark. *Structured Interview for DSM-IV Personality (SIDP-IV).* Washington, DC: American Psychiatric Press, 1997.

139. Pope, Kenneth S.; Keith-Spiegel, Patricia; and Tabachnick, Barbara G. "Sexual Attraction to Clients: The Human Therapist and the (Sometimes) Inhuman Training System." *American Psychologist* 41 (1986): 147–58.

140. Pope, Kenneth S.; Levenson, Hanna; and Schover, Leslie R. "Sexual Intimacy in Psychology Training: Results and Implications of a National Survey." *American Psychologist* 34 (1979): 682–89.

141. Quality Assurance Project. "Treatment Outlines for Paranoid, Schizotypal and Schizoid Personality Disorders." *Australian and New Zealand Journal of Psychiatry* 24 (1990): 339–50.

142. Rajagopalan, Mani; Santilli, Mario; Powell, David; Murphy, Megan; O'Brien, Marice; and Murphy, John. "Mental Health Professionals' Attire." *Australian and New Zealand Journal of Psychiatry* 32 (1998): 880–83.

143. Reich, Wilhelm. *Character Analysis.* 3d ed., enlarged. Translated by Vincent R. Carfagno. New York: Simon and Schuster, 1972.

144. Roazen, Paul. "The Problem of Silence: Training Analyses." *International Forum of Psychoanalysis* 11 (2002): 73–77.

145. Roman, Brenda, and Kay, Jerald. "Residency Education on the Prevention of Physician-Patient Sexual Misconduct." *Academic Psychiatry* 21 (1997): 26–34.

146. Rosenbaum, Max, and Muroff, Melvin, eds. *Anna O.: Fourteen Contemporary Reinterpretations.* New York: Free Press, 1984.

147. Rosenman, S. J., and Goldney, R. D. "Naming of Patients

by Therapists." *Australian and New Zealand Journal of Psychiatry* 25 (1991): 129–31.

148. Rounsaville, Bruce J.; Chevron, Eve S.; Prusoff, Brigitte A.; Elkin, Irene; Imber, Stanley; Sotsky, Stuart; and Watkins, John. "The Relation between Specific and General Dimensions of the Psychotherapy Process in Interpersonal Psychotherapy of Depression." *Journal of Consulting and Clinical Psychology* 55 (1987): 379–84.

149. Ruskin, Ronald. "Issues in Psychotherapy Supervision when Participants Are from Different Cultures." In *Clinical Perspectives on Psychotherapy Supervision,* edited by Stanley E. Greben and Ronald Ruskin, 53–72. Washington, DC: American Psychiatric Press, 1994.

150. Ryan, Christopher James. "Sex, Lies and Training Programs: The Ethics of Consensual Sexual Relationships between Psychiatrists and Trainee Psychiatrists." *Australian and New Zealand Journal of Psychiatry* 32 (1998): 387–91.

151. Ryan, William P. "Therapist's Office Is a Treatment Variable." *Psychological Reports* 45 (1979): 671–75.

152. Salzman, Leon. "Psychotherapy of the Obsessional." *American Journal of Psychotherapy* 33 (1979): 32–40.

153. Sandler, J.; Dare, C.; and Holder, A. "Basic Psychoanalytic Concepts: III. Transference." *British Journal of Psychiatry* 116 (1970): 667–72.

154. Sandler, J.; Dare, C.; and Holder, A. "Basic Psychoanalytic Concepts: IV. Counter-Transference." *British Journal of Psychiatry* 117 (1970): 83–88.

155. Sanislow, Charles A., and McGlashan, Thomas H. "Treatment Outcome of Personality Disorders." *Canadian Journal of Psychiatry* 43 (1998): 237–50.

156. Schafer, Roy. *Retelling a Life: Narration and Dialogue in Psychoanalysis.* New York: Basic Books, 1992.

157. Schwartz, Richard S., and Olds, Jacqueline. "A Phenomenology of Closeness and Its Application to Sexual Boundary Violations: A Framework for Therapists in Training." *American Journal of Psychotherapy* 56 (2002): 480–93.

158. Sederer, Lloyd I., and Libby, Mayree. "False Allegations of Sexual Misconduct: Clinical and Institutional Considerations." *Psychiatric Services* 46 (1995): 160–63.

159. Senger, Harry L. "First Name or Last? Addressing the Patient in Psychotherapy." *Comprehensive Psychiatry* 25 (1984): 38–43.

160. Shapiro, D. A. "The Effects of Therapeutic Conditions: Pos-

itive Results Revisited." *British Journal of Medical Psychology* 49 (1976): 315–23.

161. Shapiro, David. *Neurotic Styles.* New York: Basic Books, 1965.

162. Sherwood, Michael. *The Logic of Explanation in Psychoanalysis.* New York: Academic Press, 1969.

163. Simon, Robert I. "Commentary: Treatment Boundaries—Flexible Guidelines, not Rigid Standards." *Journal of the American Academy of Psychiatry and the Law* 29 (2001): 287–89.

164. Simon, Robert I. "Sexual Exploitation of Patients: How It Begins Before It Happens." *Psychiatric Annals* 19 (1989): 104–12.

165. Simon, Robert I. "Therapist-Patient Sex: From Boundary Violations to Sexual Misconduct." *Psychiatric Clinics of North America* 22 (1999): 31–47.

166. Slavney, Phillip R. *Perspectives on "Hysteria."* Baltimore: Johns Hopkins University Press, 1990.

167. Slavney, Phillip R., and McHugh, Paul R. "Life-Stories and Meaningful Connections: Reflections on a Clinical Method in Psychiatry and Medicine." *Perspectives in Biology and Medicine* 27 (1984): 279–88.

168. Sloane, R. Bruce; Cristol, Allan H.; Pepernik, Max C.; and Staples, Fred R. "Role Preparation and Expectation of Improvement in Psychotherapy." *Journal of Nervous and Mental Disease* 150 (1970): 18–26.

169. Spence, Donald P. *Narrative Truth and Historical Truth: Meaning and Interpretation in Psychoanalysis.* New York: W. W. Norton, 1982.

170. Strupp, Hans H. "The Performance of Psychiatrists and Psychologists in a Therapeutic Interview." *Journal of Clinical Psychology* 14 (1958): 219–26.

171. Summergrad, Paul; Herman, John B.; Weilburg, Jeffrey B.; and Jellinek, Michael S. "Wagons Ho: Forward on the Managed Care Trail." *General Hospital Psychiatry* 17 (1995): 251–59.

172. Tickle, Jennifer J.; Heatherton, Todd F.; and Wittenberg, Lauren G. "Can Personality Change?" In *Handbook of Personality Disorders: Theory, Research, and Treatment,* edited by W. John Livesley, 242–58. New York: Guilford Press, 2001.

173. Truax, Charles B., and Carkhuff, Robert R. *Toward Effective Counseling and Psychotherapy: Training and Practice.* Chicago: Aldine, 1967.

174. Truax, Charles B.; Wargo, Donald G.; Frank, Jerome D.; Imber, Stanley D.; Battle, Carolyn C.; Hoehn-Saric, Rudolf; Nash, Earl H.; and Stone, Anthony R. "Therapist Empathy, Genuineness, and Warmth and Patient Therapeutic Outcome." *Journal of Consulting Psychology* 30 (1966): 395–401.

175. Uhlenhuth, E. H., and Duncan, David B. "Subjective Change with Medical Student Therapists: I. Course of Relief in Psychoneurotic Outpatients." *Archives of General Psychiatry* 18 (1968): 428–38.

176. Uhlenhuth, E. H., and Duncan, David B. "Subjective Change with Medical Student Therapists: II. Some Determinants of Change in Psychoneurotic Outpatients." *Archives of General Psychiatry* 18 (1968): 532–40.

177. Vamos, Marina. "The Concept of Appropriate Professional Boundaries in Psychiatric Practice: A Pilot Training Course." *Australian and New Zealand Journal of Psychiatry* 35 (2001): 613–18.

178. Voglmaier, Martina M.; Seidman, Larry J.; Niznikiewicz, Margaret A.; Dickey, Chandlee C.; Shenton, Martha E.; and McCarley, Robert W. "Verbal and Nonverbal Neuropsychological Test Performance in Subjects with Schizotypal Personality Disorder." *American Journal of Psychiatry* 157 (2000): 787–93.

179. Voglmaier, Martina M.; Seidman, Larry J.; Salisbury, Dean; and McCarley, Robert W. "Neuropsychological Dysfunction in Schizotypal Personality Disorder: A Profile Analysis." *Biological Psychiatry* 41 (1997): 530–40.

180. Weiner, Myron F. "Personal Openness with Patients: Help or Hindrance." *Texas Medicine* 76 (1980): 60–62.

181. Weintraub, Daniel; Dixon, Lisa; Kohlhepp, Elizabeth; and Woolery, Janet. "Residents in Personal Psychotherapy: A Longitudinal and Cross-Sectional Perspective." *Academic Psychiatry* 23 (1999): 14–19.

182. Weissman, Sidney. "American Psychiatry in the 21st Century: The Discipline, Its Practice, and Its Work Force." *Bulletin of the Menninger Clinic* 58 (1994): 502–18.

183. Widiger, Thomas A. "Categorical versus Dimensional Classification: Implications from and for Research." *Journal of Personality Disorders* 6 (1992): 287–300.

184. Wilbers, D.; Veenstra, G.; van de Wiel, H. B. M.; and Weijmar Schultz, W. C. M. "Sexual Contact in the Doctor-Patient Relationship in the Netherlands." *British Medical Journal* 304 (1992): 1531–34.

185. Williams, Chris, and Whitfield, Graeme. "Written and

Computer-Based Self-Help Treatments for Depression." *British Medical Bulletin* 57 (2001): 133–44.

186. Wolberg, Lewis R. *The Technique of Psychotherapy.* 4th ed. 2 vols. Orlando, FL: Grune and Stratton, 1988.

187. Yager, Joel; Docherty, John P.; and Tischler, Gary L. "Preparing Psychiatric Residents for Managed Care: Values, Proficiencies, Curriculum, and Implications for Psychotherapy Training." *Journal of Psychotherapy Practice and Research* 6 (1997): 108–22.

188. Yeung, Albert S.; Lyons, Michael J.; Waternaux, Christine M.; Faraone, Stephen V.; and Tsuang, Ming T. "The Relationship between DSM-III Personality Disorders and the Five-Factor Model of Personality." *Comprehensive Psychiatry* 34 (1993): 227–34.

189. Zimmerman, Mark; Pfohl, Bruce; Stangl, Dalene; and Corenthal, Caryn. "Assessment of DSM-III Personality Disorders: The Importance of Interviewing an Informant." *Journal of Clinical Psychiatry* 47 (1986): 261–63.

190. Zur, Ofer, and Lazarus, Arnold A. "Six Arguments against Dual Relationships and Their Rebuttals." In *Dual Relationships and Psychotherapy,* edited by Arnold A. Lazarus and Ofer Zur, 3–24. New York: Springer, 2002.

Index

32–33, 41–42. *See also* NEO Personality Inventory, Revised; Personality; Structured Interview for DSM-IV Personality

Transference, 54, 70–71, 74, 75, 78, 91

Truax, Charles, 66

Uhlenhuth, E. H., 60–61

Weintraub, Daniel, 52–53
Weissman, Sidney, 53
Woodward, Christel, 82–83

Zur, Ofer, 80

Phillip R. Slavney, M.D., is the Eugene Meyer III Professor of Psychiatry and Medicine at the Johns Hopkins University School of Medicine. He was Director of Residency Education in the Department of Psychiatry and Behavioral Sciences at the Oregon Health and Science University from 1974 to 1976 and was Director of Residency Education in the Department of Psychiatry and Behavioral Sciences at the Johns Hopkins University School of Medicine from 1977 to 1993. Dr. Slavney has been a psychotherapy supervisor for more than thirty years, has published articles on psychotherapy for beginners, and is co-author with Paul R. McHugh of *The Perspectives of Psychiatry*, now in its second edition.